In the Freedom of Space

Margaret Comin

Copyright © 2024 Margaret Comin

All rights reserved.

ISBN: 979-8989695324

Dedication

To my beloved husband, Bill, who has always stood by me.

~*~

*"I called to the Lord from my narrow prison;
He answered me in the freedom of space."* Psalm 118

Contents

Chapter One	1
Chapter Two	12
Chapter Three	17
Chapter Four	27
Chapter Five	35
Chapter Six	47
Chapter Seven	71
Chapter Eight	93
Chapter Nine	103
Chapter Ten	123
Chapter Eleven	149
Chapter Twelve	153
Chapter Thirteen	158

Acknowledgments

To our wonderful children, Meredith and Douglas, thank you for your constant love and support.

To my big brother, William (Billy), thank you for always holding me to a higher standard.

To my sisters: Nancy, Jan and Tacy—thanks for always being so lovely.

To my nieces, Emily and Betsy, and my nephew Andy—thanks for your ongoing interest in my book.

To Tony Grooms, a fabulous professor of creative writing, and to Linda Nieman, a great professor of memoir writing, thanks again. And finally, to Josh Langston, my wonderful editor and publisher.

Peggy

Chapter One

The Now

We stood in my mother's living room and she said, "I'm getting in bed, Peg-a-roo. Fix me a ham and cheese sandwich on rye with mayonnaise, some potato chips, and a cup of coffee. Bring them to me in bed. I've had a stomachache all day, but I just took my temperature and it's ninety-eight point six."

I was sixty years old, and I had flown into Jacksonville, Florida, the day before to visit my 86-year-old mother in her new cottage in a retirement center. My husband Bill couldn't come with me because he had to work. I was totally blind in my right eye and had only light perception and the ability to see the color red in my left. My mother kept her place very darkened, and I couldn't see a thing. I had no idea where the refrigerator was, let alone the ham, the cheese, the rye bread, the mayonnaise or the instant coffee. I thought the kitchen was on my right, which turned out to be true, and I located a stove with a pot, a cup, and a jar of instant coffee on it. (Momma had never owned a teakettle.) Feeling around carefully, I found a spigot and filled the pot halfway to the top with water. No grime floated to the top, so I found a burner eye, placed the pot on it, and turned on the stove. A whirring sound led me to the refrigerator, and I opened the door and felt around for the ham, the cheese, and the mayonnaise. I turned around and almost bumped into the kitchen table, where I smelled a loaf of rye bread.

Momma always had places set at her table, so I touched around until I found a placemat, then grabbed a table knife for the mayonnaise and a spoon for the coffee. Somehow, I found some paper plates and paper napkins on the counter and proceeded to make the sandwich.

Hearing the water at a full boil, I walked to the stove, grabbed the pot and turned off the burner. The idea of pouring boiling water into a cup and using the tip of my index finger as a fill guide made me anxious, but there it was.

"Where's your cat?" I called to Momma. If the cat was inside, I had to be careful not to trip over her.

"Outside," Momma called back.

I decided to take the plate of food first. I had heard Momma walk through the door of the bedroom after she originally asked me for the sandwich, so I had a good idea where the bedroom door was. "Momma?" I called. "Which bed are you in?"

"On your right," she said as I entered. "Looks delicious, darling."

I handed her the plate, walked back into the kitchen, and stirred the coffee. I had always heard that if you didn't look down at a cup of coffee you were carrying, it wouldn't spill. I didn't have that problem.

"I'll take it," Momma said from her sitting position on the bed. "Hooray, Peg-a-roo," she said. Then, "Maybe I can read you some of *Green Mansions* while you are here."

She knew I couldn't stand that book about that bird girl. We both started laughing. "How about *David Copperfield* or *A Tale of Two Cities*?" she continued.

"Does *A Tale of Two Cities* start with the line, 'It was the best of times, it was the worst of times,'" I asked.

"Yes," Momma said, "and it is a wonderful story."

"I like Dickens better than *Green Mansions*," I said. I'd forgotten her potato chips, and rose to get them. "Your potato chips!" I exclaimed. Then I continued, "But I don't like Dickens very much. I imagine you don't have a copy of *East of Eden* or *The Grapes of Wrath*, Momma?"

"You know I heartily dislike Steinbeck," she said. "Well, I recently had a poem published in the retirement-center magazine," she said. "It was called 'On Envy.' I'll read it to you in a minute. Out of five hundred residents here nobody even commented on it. Don't you like some recognition?"

"Yes, Momma."

"You know that nice lady who lives here and lost use of her hands? She is such a good sport. I feed her dinner on Sunday night. She can't even hold a magazine and read it. Besides, her grown son recently died. I don't see how people stand things like that."

I didn't either. Sometimes Momma would say things like *it's not what happens to you but the way you take it,* but that was as far as she'd go.

I found the chips next to the plates and napkins. Typical of Momma—the bag was open and the chips were soft and stale. Sometimes Momma left a gallon of milk on the counter until it was sour and useless. I wouldn't have been surprised if I went back into the refrigerator and encountered some moldy food. I washed my hands and filled a napkin with potato chips. The cat meowed at the front door. I didn't want to let her in.

Momma must have turned on her Sirius radio because it sounded like a Beethoven symphony was playing forth. I stood still for a moment. I wondered how Momma had handled my blindness without ever really saying how difficult it was for her.

***

I suppose that day in Houston in 1955 began like any other. My brother, Billy, age four, and I, age two and a half, would have bounded out of bed early. I understand that, on this particular day, Billy went to a playmate's house. As usual, Daddy would have driven off to work as a geologist at an oil well for Shell. I'm sure I watched his car as he backed down the driveway. He always honked as he turned onto the street.

Later that morning, Momma said, she was reading to me on the fluffy gray sofa in the living room. She said I had refused to change out of my pink nightgown and insisted on wearing my red rubber rain boots even though it was a sunny day. She read from *A Child's Garden of Verses:* "I'm hiding, I'm hiding, and no one knows where / For all they can see are my toes and my hair."

The doorbell rang. I jumped up and ran to the door in my red rubber rain boots and opened it. Our cocker spaniel, Snowy, flew to the door with me, barking fiercely. Snowy shot right on outside. "Hooray, it's the plumber! He's going to fix the kitchen sink," Momma said. "I didn't know I wasn't supposed to pour hot grease down the kitchen sink. By the way, I'm Mary Jean Paul, and this is Peggy."

"I'm Mark," the plumber said.

I ran ahead as Momma and the plumber walked to the kitchen. She started ironing. She said she burned a hole with the iron in one of Daddy's shirts. It seemed definite that she didn't iron well. She was a former debutante and had been raised with servants who cooked, cleaned and ironed. She said once that she never realized she'd have to wash dishes when she married. She thought servants or fairies would do them. While Momma ironed, I played near her feet. The clogged sink had some standing water in it. The plumber took out a can of what we now know was Red Devil Lye, poured the crystals into the water and started plunging.

Research tells us that modern drain cleaners, like Drano, consist of around 40% sodium hydroxide or lye—an alkaline substance that is extremely caustic. At the 40% concentration, which dissolves grease and hair in clogged pipes, Drano and similar products can cause serious chemical burns, especially on mucous membranes. Higher concentrations are difficult to purchase nowadays, in part because they are extremely dangerous, and in part because sodium hydroxide is used to manufacture crystal meth.

Red Devil Lye, which is no longer manufactured, was 100% sodium hydroxide. As the lye crystals dissolved in the sink, the water began bubbling with heat. Mark worked the plunger, splashing the water all the way to the rim of the sink. Just as he gave a vigorous plunge, I dashed over to see what he was doing. He didn't see me. I looked up at him just as a wave of caustic liquid lye splashed out of the sink, striking my eyes.

I almost passed out from the pain. I screamed and screamed. Neither my mother nor father ever talked much about that day in later years.

The plumber took Momma and me in his truck to the hospital. Momma tried to hold and comfort me as I screamed and as the plumber drove his speeding truck, tools rattling in the bed, to the emergency room.

My father met us there. The doctors put me on morphine and told my parents my corneas had been severely burned and that I would most likely be blind. They said it would be quite a while before I could even open my eyes.

When I was able to open my eyes, the doctors said my left eye was badly damaged, and any surgery would be a longshot. They said the right eye was destroyed and would need a prosthesis later on.

I don't remember being in the hospital in Houston. Momma later said she brought me a toy every day. She also said once that sometimes people give presents out of guilt.

When I was older, I would learn that Mark, the plumber, was young. Momma, however, was twenty-eight years old. Daddy once said that if Momma had been another kind of woman, the accident would never have happened. Daddy's mother and sisters were pragmatic New Englanders. I think that they or my practical Midwestern friend Barbara represented the kind of woman he meant.

Barbara was Momma's age. She said that when her kids were young, in the early 1950s, the mere sight of the Red Devil Lye can with the picture of the big red devil made her send her kids outside.

***

"Any chance of my potato chips?" Momma called.

"Oh, sorry," I said. "I just got bogged down in my own thoughts."

"Isn't this Beethoven just beautiful?" Momma asked.

"Sure," I said as I made my way into her bedroom and tried to focus on the sounds of the orchestra coming from the Sirius radio.

I handed Momma the paper napkin full of potato chips. "You're a sweetheart," she said.

I sprawled on the extra twin bed. "Brahms is next," she cried. "I am so glad I can still play some Beethoven, Brahms, and Chopin on the piano."

The silent tension between my mother and me has always been this: she could have picked me up and prevented my blindness. True, she was accustomed to servants watching children and servants ironing. But the fact was, she didn't have any servants, and I was two and a half.

We never talked about this. Ever.

Irresponsibility and poor judgment go hand in hand. Momma showed both in her lifetime. Like when she was a senior in high school and she and her friend Arvilla sat across the street from their principal's office the last week of school, smoking cigarettes in Arvilla's parked car. The principal expelled both girls, but Momma's daddy, a lawyer, got her reinstated so she could graduate. Arvilla didn't get to graduate. She was killed the next week while speeding down the road.

And what about my mother's depression? How depressed was she the day I was blinded? Did irresponsibility, poor judgment and depression play into it?

***

It was freezing in this bedroom. I wanted to say something to Momma about it but decided against it. Momma always turned the thermostat down, no matter what month it was. I tried to wrap myself up in the lightweight bedspread. "Thank you, darling, for the lunch," she said.

"You're welcome," I said.

"I have a joke," Momma said over the sound of the music.

"A man and his wife stopped in Kissimmee, Florida, on a road trip."

"The woman pursed her lips and said, 'So where are we?'"

"'Stopped for lunch,' the man said."

"'I know, but where?' the woman asked."

"'On our road trip,' the man said."

"'I know but where are we?'" the woman asked, hoping he would say Kissimmee.

"Burger King!" The man replied.

Momma laughed uproariously, and I laughed some. When our laughter subsided, she said, "Music makes me feel better. A friend is coming by in a little while to play some duets. I think you'll like her. And everybody admires you."

"Thank you," I said.

She would say that much, but she wouldn't talk with me about the accident. I wish she would tell me every single detail of that day. One of her friends had told me Momma talked about my accident sometimes, and that she had a lot of guilt. I asked my brother, Billy, if I should just bring it up with her. "Only if you want a major fight on your hands," he said.

Then my brother said: "Piglet, I'm surprised you're not over that whole blinding thing by now."

I had to laugh. I know my brother really admires me.

I used to wonder in what month I was blinded. Momma finally said it was in May. I asked her what day in May. She said she had purposely forgotten. So, I was blinded in the beauty of spring. I wish I could see all the flowers.

Momma broke into my thoughts. "I'm just so jealous of everybody here. Florence is an angel because she does for everybody. Mary Ruth is a superstar because she grew up in a Japanese internment camp. Erma is president of everything. I think I'm going crazy, and I need my hair done, and I need new clothes."

"Momma, do you still read the Bible for one hour every morning?"

"Oh, yes. I love the Bible. My favorite book of the Old Testament is Psalms, and my favorite book of the New Testament is the gospel of Matthew."

"Momma, I came across the writings of Viktor Frankl, the psychoanalyst and author who was imprisoned at Auschwitz for three years. He had tremendous faith and marvelous insights. One insight I love is: 'When all other freedoms are lost, we have one freedom left: the freedom to choose our own attitude.'"

"That is beautiful," Momma said. "By the way, I hear Jenny meowing at the back door. Can you let her in? It opens right into the back of my bedroom."

When I opened the door, it looked light outside. I managed to get Jenny into the bedroom.

I wanted to ask Momma about the cat. My daughter had said the cat was way overweight and Momma let her graze all day long. The vet wanted the cat to eat once a day. If Momma went into assisted living it would be hard for her to give up the cat.

**

I couldn't stop thinking about my blinding. My father sued the plumbing company in 1955, and the plumber was found at fault. Settlements were low in the 1950s and most of mine was used for experimental eye surgery in New York. My parents took me to Columbia University Hospital to see one of the most internationally renowned corneal surgeons. His name was Ramon Castroviejo. He had limited success with corneal transplants in the 1950s. They usually failed after a short while. This was because there were no steroids then, and immunosuppression had not been discovered.

I don't know much about New York, except sometimes I would see some in my left eye after a surgery. But then, adults would say the corneal transplant had rejected. And I would go blind again. I was terrified, and I didn't understand. What did it do psychologically to a young child to see and not to see and see again and not see?

My right eye was enucleated, so nothing could be done for it.

My father disappeared from New York not long after the surgeries started, so Clara, my grandmother's cook, took the train to New York to stay with Momma in a hotel. I went back and forth from the hotel to the hospital.

Clara told me later it was a bad time, but "that was life, and we couldn't help it."

Momma told me later it made her feel better that the plumber was found at fault. She seemed to believe this story proved something, but I really didn't. Who was really responsible?

About 20 years ago, when I was 40, I got an interesting phone call from Billy. He said he had just seen a legal document on Momma's desk referring to a lawsuit with the plumbing company. Momma came up behind him and asked him to get her a glass of water. He left to get it and when he came back, the document was gone.

Before Daddy died in 1992, I wondered if he would have told me anything about the eye injury. I never asked him. He was always married to some subsequent wife. Not that Daddy was great-looking or anything. He had brown hair and small blue eyes and a medium build.

***

Thunderous applause came across the Sirius radio as the Brahms symphony ended. "I wish my mother had appreciated my love of music," Momma said.

I was freezing but didn't want to say so. I wondered where the thermostat was in this place. But then again, would I try to change the temp even if I could and risk Momma's annoyance?

"My mother criticized me in so many ways," Momma continued. "Not only in my love of music. If I practiced on the piano, it bothered her. When I was older, sometimes she blew up and yelled that I should be out at a Junior League meeting or a Colonial Dames meeting."

The phone rang. "It's probably my neighbor Dee," Momma said. "I hate her. She calls me three and four times a day to see what I am doing. And sometimes I have Johnny pick me up at the back so she won't see me leaving. If he picks me up at the front, she always asks me where Johnny has driven me in Jacksonville. He has just dropped me off at the Yacht Club to meet friends for lunch or taken me to the doctor or on errands, but I don't want to talk about it. Would you want someone knowing where you were going all the time?"

Johnny worked as a driver for Momma and several other people.

"Probably not," I said. "But you've always really liked your privacy. When I was a child, I remember you wanted uninterrupted blocks of time. And you said it bothered you that your mother always asked you everything you did when you went out on dates."

"The only thing my mother ever said I did right was put butter on saltine crackers for a snack. She'd put them in the oven and toast them. We only did this on Clara's day off, but she said I put the right amount of butter on the crackers."

"And you correct me too, Peggy. I can't stand it when you sometimes ask me if the milk has expired. You're much harder on me than your brother is!"

The phone started ringing again. "I'm not answering it," Momma said. "I'm sure it is Dee."

I felt sorry for my mother. Very sorry.

***

The other day, Bill Googled "Red Devil Lye" for me, and it was mainly an interesting review.

1. Red Devil Lye is no longer manufactured.
2. It was used as a drain cleaner.
3. It was used in the making of soap.
4. It was caustic and hazardous to eyes.
5. Both sides in World War II used Red Devil Lye in the manufacturing of methamphetamine, which was given to troops to keep them awake.

***

My mother has not mentioned my blindness in more than 40 years. She does sometimes mention my one prosthetic eye.

I'm not sure she ever fully accepted my blindness. But she

provided me with some very interesting experiences and allowed me some unusual freedoms. Like every morning in the summer, Momma let me leave home at 10:00 AM, and she told me to be home by 6:00 PM.

My father looked down on me because of my disability. If I said, "It's a pretty day," he said, "How do you know? You can't see."

Then I felt terrible.

I think my mother loved my father initially. She grew up in Jacksonville, Florida, and he grew up in New York and Massachusetts. Her father was a successful lawyer, and her parents had been married for thirty-two years. Dad's father vanished when Dad was four years old, and he was raised by very wealthy and indulgent foster parents. Mother's friend John Rogers from Jacksonville, was Dad's roommate at Harvard, and he had introduced Mother and Dad. She was studying at the Boston Conservatory of Music. Dad and Mother used to go on picnics near Plymouth Rock. Mother was more honest. She told Dad how she hated her mother, and how she hated being a debutante. Dad was honest about all his accolades from the Colorado School of Mines. He had awards to prove them. However, he told Mother he had given up drinking (he had not), and that he would go to church with her forever. He only went to church during their engagement.

Mother and Dad dreamed of being African explorers. Unfortunately, when Mother married him, it was either an irresponsible act or an error in judgment. Dad turned out to be an alcoholic, a loser, and perhaps mentally ill.

Doctors tell me there is no visual memory before the age of three. All I could see, after the accident, was light, dark and the color red in one eye and nothing in the other. On that fateful day, I know I was wearing a pink nightgown and red rubber rain boots. But what was Momma wearing? And what was the plumber wearing? I guess the last things I ever saw were our kitchen in Houston, Momma at an ironing board, and the plumber at the sink.

How did Momma stand walking into that kitchen again? Can you imagine standing in a room where your child was permanently blinded and disfigured for life?

In all the chaos of my childhood, Momma certainly showed much love to me. She said things like: "You're beautiful, peach cake" or "You and your brother are the two best things that ever happened to me!"

The disfigurement of my face has been almost as difficult as my blindness. My injured right eye appeared all white but with red lines in it. The idea that my face might have been attractive with two normal eyes has always haunted me. My girlfriend Laurie says I have never had beautiful features, so I would never have been beautiful anyway.

People have always remarked to me that my mother is (or at least was) beautiful. She had beautiful high cheekbones and beautiful blue eyes. Apparently, she was the most gorgeous of all the debutantes. It has become very tiresome. Even Billy says Momma was a knockout when she was young. Mom is now eighty-six, and people say, *"Your mom looks great!"* Yet of all people, my mother couldn't have cared less that she was or is beautiful. Of course, she wanted her hair done, and she wanted nice clothes, but that was all.

My husband always says I looked very pretty, but the well of insecurity runs too deep. Too many kids made hateful comments from kindergarten through the fifth grade.

Sometimes, when I think about my disfigurement and my disability, I think about Elizabeth Smith and her story. In 1983, Elizabeth, age 6, dashed out of her house in Atlanta and went out to play in several inches of snow. She touched a downed power line. Firemen were supposed to be watching the line. Eventually, gangrene set in for Elizabeth. She lost both arms and one leg.

Our stories are similar. Two blonde, blue-eyed girls dash forth into disaster.

Chapter Two

Billy was five and I was three when we were riding on the hood of Momma's Willys station wagon. The hood ornament, really a simple strip of chrome, was between us. We hung on to the strip as Momma drove through the evening countryside. "There goes a jackrabbit," Billy said.

"I wish I could see a jackrabbit," I said. Then I asked, "Do you see any stars tonight?"

"Yes," Billy said. "'Star light, star bright, first star I see tonight, I wish I may, I wish I might have the wish I wish tonight.' I wish my sister Peggy could see again."

"Y'all doing okay out there?" Momma called through the open window.

"Yes," we called back.

If I tried hard, I could see the headlights of the Willys shining on the road in front.

I find it amazing that Momma had a blind three-year-old riding on the front of her car as she drove down a country road. I mentioned that to Billy not long ago and he said, "What about me?"

What happens to a normal child when a sibling becomes seriously disabled? I believe that I, the injured child, was brought to the forefront. Momma went with me to Boston and New York for experimental surgeries in the mid-1950s while Billy was shuffled off to relatives. Billy didn't see Momma for a whole year. Still, as a child, I always thought that Billy didn't suffer. After all, he could run fast and jump high and read and print in kindergarten, what other help did he need? As an adult, I know he did suffer during those years.

When Billy could see the stars and I could not, the separateness and the closeness of our lives began.

***

When I was three, I remember wearing a Trundle Bundle on cold winter nights. I hated it. Daddy put me in it, because one night I was wandering around the house after my bedtime and got in bed with him and Momma. I had to sit on the side of my bed while Daddy put my feet in the Trundle Bundle, and then he told me to stand up while he zipped it from my ankle to my neck. Zzzzip! The feet had rubber padding but the legs weren't cut up very high, so I was forced to walk slowly: I was sort of in a sack. The Trundle Bundle had long sleeves so I could move my arms all around. "I don't like this thing," I said to Billy, who was in his twin bed across the room.

"I wouldn't like it either," he said. "I don't have to wear one. Besides, that thing is pink."

I told Momma I hated wearing the Trundle Bundle! She said she would rather I slept in pajamas so I could get around easily, but Daddy was the man of the house, and we had to follow his wishes. So I climbed in bed in my Trundle Bundle on cold Texas nights and put my thumb in my mouth and stared at the darkness.

"You don't have to sleep in that thing when it gets hot," Billy said.

When I was older, I realized Daddy wanted Momma in bed to himself.

***

Momma and I went to church one Sunday when I was four. She told me to stay in the nursery. The children in the nursery were crying, and I started to cry. A man who smelled like Daddy and cigars carried me into the church and sat me beside Momma. It was cold in the church, and I snuggled up to her soft mink coat.

The organ began to play, and I sat quietly in the pew. Momma stood to sing. *"Oh, Jesus, I have promised,"* Momma sang out. I knew these words, because Momma sang them every day.

After church, Momma took me by the hand. "Five steps down," she said outside, and I carefully held her hand and counted the five steps down. They were concrete.

We kept turning corners. I put out my other hand and felt the bricks of the church building. Suddenly Momma stopped and said, "You should have stayed in the nursery. I wanted to be by myself in church to listen to the sermon and read the Bible without interruption."

Momma grabbed me then and spanked me very hard. I was so surprised. As time went on I experienced other rages with Momma. They weren't frequent, and usually she would become extremely quiet before they happened. If she fell silent and then said, "Peggy," in a certain tone of voice, I knew it was time to leave the room. The night of my spanking after church, Momma read Billy and me extra books. We liked *Ginger Pickles, Rikki-Tikki-Tavi, and A Child's Garden of Verses*. Momma read us books to apologize for spankings.

***

I was still four when Daddy bought a statue of a lady and put it on the sideboard in the dining room of our house in Houston. He said it was made of marble and that I was not to touch it. I had no interest in the statue. I loved my toys, which were in the bottom of the sideboard. I had my Tiny Tears doll. Her eyes were perfect. They opened the same amount. Not like mine. I also had a top. I could put the top on the floor and start spinning it but then when it spun away from me I couldn't find it.

One day Daddy said I could hold the statue and feel it. He said, "I want you to do that, Peep-eye, and I want you to feel it."

The nickname never bothered me. My Dad had called me Peep-eye since before I was blind. He would hold his newspaper in front of his face and then lower it and call, *Peep-eye!*

The statue felt hard and smooth. "Those are her breasts," Daddy said as I felt two round bumps on the front of the statue. "Momma has breasts," I said.

"She sure does. Nice ones," Daddy said.

Then I felt the statue's hair, which was hard. Her arms and legs were long. I reached up and felt her eyes. They opened the same amount.

"What color is your statue, Daddy?" I asked.

"White," he said.

The next day Momma said it was Thanksgiving Day. Billy and I were sitting at the dining-room table playing Rock, Paper, Scissors. I felt the sun streaming in on my arms and face. Momma said she would be serving Thanksgiving dinner soon on her beautiful plates with a different bird on each one. She said I would have the scissortail flycatcher and Billy would have the Canadian jay.

"I smelled that funny smell on Daddy again today," Billy said.

"You did?" I asked.

"Somebody said it's from drinking whiskey," Billy said.

It was a strange smell. I wondered what whiskey was. Sometimes Daddy smelled like cigars.

Suddenly I heard Daddy's footsteps in the dining room and the shattering of glass. "Daddy just threw that marble statue through the window!" Billy exclaimed.

Billy grabbed me by the arm, and we both were shaking. Then he released my arm and said, "It broke all over the driveway. Daddy is out there sweeping up statue pieces and the glass from the window. I don't understand this at all."

Momma came in from the kitchen. "I guess you children are all right, I am just going to go ahead and serve lunch. Please sit at your places at the table."

I was scared. What did Daddy do that for?

As an adult, one day when Momma seemed approachable, I asked her if I remembered this statue story correctly. She said I did. I asked Billy if he remembered it, and he said, "Not at all."

***

On a warm day shortly after Thanksgiving, I outsmarted Billy. He was six, and I was four. We both loved to climb the tree in our front yard in Houston. We were up in the tree. "Hey," Billy said, "Take off your shorts and underwear and give them to me. I'll throw them on the ground and you can climb down and get them. After that, I'll take off my shorts and underwear and give them to you, and you can throw them on the ground, and I'll climb down and get them."

"You go first," I said.

He handed me his shorts and underwear, and I threw them to the ground. I heard his feet crackling the bark and then thudding to the ground when he jumped. "I'm dressed and coming back up," he yelled.

Oh, no, I thought. And then I said, "My turn, I'm going in the house. I'll be right back."

I climbed down the tree and ran in the house to the room Billy and I shared. I felt on a chair and found a dress. I threw off my shorts and shirt and put on the dress. Then I ran outside and climbed carefully up the tree. It wasn't very easy in a dress. I sat on the branch beside Billy. I pulled off my underwear and gave it to him. "Throw it down," I shouted, and stuck out my tongue.

If Momma noticed this game, she never said anything to Billy or me about it.

***

One day when I was five and Billy was seven, Daddy took us to see an oil well. He worked in Texas because of the 1950's oil boom.

Daddy talked to me about different kinds of minerals as we walked toward the well. I began to cough because of the strong smell of oil. Daddy stopped and didn't let me go any further. "What does it look like?" I asked.

Riding home in the car, Billy suggested a game of Animal, Vegetable or Mineral. "Let me go first," I cried.

"Is it an animal, vegetable or mineral, peep-eye?" Daddy asked.

"Mineral," I said as I felt the car pick up speed. The wind blew harder through the open window.

Billy and Daddy didn't even have a chance to guess.

"It's shale!" I cried.

"You are smart!" Daddy exclaimed.

My daddy thought I was smart. I felt great. I knew I could do anything if my daddy thought I was smart. To this day I cherish this compliment. Daddy was super-smart, although his career was ruined by his drinking and possibly some kind of mental-health issue. But when I was five years old, he said I was smart.

Chapter Three

"Momma said she and Daddy are getting a divorce," seven-year-old Billy said.

"What does that mean?" I asked.

"There's a kid in second grade who said his parents are getting a divorce," Billy said. "His father left, and he just lives with his mother."

"Why are Momma and Daddy getting a divorce?"

"I heard Momma say Daddy just lost another job, and he drinks all the time."

We were sitting on Billy's twin bed in our room. I felt the satiny-smooth headboard. I had a matching bed and Momma told me the wood parts of it were brown.

"Who would we live with?" I asked.

"Momma said we would go live with her and our grandparents in Florida," Billy said.

"I'm scared of Daddy. He bought me a doll stroller and I ran it into a new chair and ripped the—what do you call that stuff that covers a chair?"

"Upholstery," Billy said, sounding important.

"Well, he yelled at me. Loud. I think Momma is a lot nicer than Daddy."

"So do I," Billy said.

In 1959 very few people got divorced. If they did, the person seeking the divorce had to have a good reason. Daddy separated from Momma a few years after my accident, but it was Momma who ultimately sought the divorce. For years I didn't know what the formal grounds for divorce were. In 1984, right before her death, Grandmomma said to Billy, "We had tapes."

Grandmomma was very exacting about detail.

"Tapes of what?" Billy asked.

"Tapes of your father with other women."

"What?" Billy asked in astonishment.

"Your grandfather hired a detective to follow your father around, and the detective taped your father with other women. So, the grounds for divorce were infidelity."

Our father's marriage to Momma was the first of four.

***

When Momma left Daddy, she and Billy and I took a taxi to the airport to fly to Jacksonville to live with our grandparents. I loved Granddaddy, because he read me chapters in *The Bobbsey Twins and Baby May*. I was scared of Grandmomma because if I said "Yes" instead of "Yes Ma'am," she clapped her hands loudly at me.

As I climbed the steep steps of the plane, I felt my velvet hat blow away. It was my favorite hat.

"I'll get it," Billy yelled, and he ran back down the steps.

"It sure is windy," Momma said.

Billy clattered back up the steps and put the hat in my hand.

Soon after we got to Jacksonville, Billy and I were sitting on a bed in our grandmother's front bedroom. He started to describe the room. "This room has eight windows and two walls," he said. "It has a fireplace with another fireplace just below it in the living room. They share a chimney. Grandmother has Oriental rugs in this bedroom, and they are really old."

"Peggy, Billy, come eat your supper," called my grandmother's cook, Clara.

Billy ran down the stairs toward the front hallway with me in hot pursuit. I counted five familiar steps to a landing, thirteen more familiar steps to another landing, then three final steps to the hallway. I made my way to the sitting room and felt for my TV tray, then felt for my place on the sofa to sit with the tray in front of me. Clara always served us on TV trays with newspaper underneath to catch any spills. "I'm putting the paper under your TV tray right now," Clara said, and I heard the newspaper crinkle.

I smelled fried chicken, and in a moment Clara put a plate on my tray. "You have fried chicken, rice and gravy, squash and string beans and a hot biscuit all buttered. Don't that sound good, darlin'? Now I'm gonna go get Billy's."

"Oh, go on, Billy," Clara said, and I knew he had just jumped up and untied her apron as she was leaving the room. This was a common Billy trick.

Billy and I ate in silence. I could hear my grandmother's voice in my head saying, "Chew with your mouth closed."

My favorite part of supper was dessert. "Here's your vanilla ice cream with chocolate sauce," Clara said. "The spoon is in the bowl on your right."

"Thank you, Clara," I said. I stirred my vanilla ice cream and chocolate sauce together until I had soup.

"Grandmomma said I have to go to kindergarten," I said. I directed this at my brother, at the other end of the sofa.

"Kindergarten is easy," Billy said.

"Grandmomma and Granddaddy want me to go to the School for the Blind in St. Augustine, but Momma wants me to go to school with sighted kids."

"You have to color pictures in kindergarten," Billy said. "That might be hard for you."

"I can see red," I said.

"But there are a lot of other colors. Like there are green and yellow and orange and blue and purple and brown."

One day Grandmomma had shown me different colors of construction paper. I could only pick out the one that was red. She named all the other colors but I couldn't see any differences between them.

"You have to start raising your hand in kindergarten," Billy said. "I'll show you later how you're supposed to hold up your hand." That was good, because I didn't know how to raise my hand, how high to raise it or whether to hold it way high in the air, or wave it, or just what to do.

***

Momma, Billy and I were all living in with Grandmomma and Granddaddy in their house. Momma stayed in her room, the middle bedroom, most of the time. When I went to visit her, I could tell the room was very dark, even in the daytime. It smelled like cigarettes.

Grandmomma took me for my first day of kindergarten. I wore a new dress. Grandmomma said it was pink and made of cotton. Clara starched and ironed it for me, and when I put it on she buttoned it up the back. She said I looked pretty. Mrs. Brooks, the kindergarten teacher, took me by the hand and walked me to a table. I bumped into the corner of the table, but it didn't hurt. One of the great frustrations of blindness is walking into things. Not only do we sometimes hurt ourselves, it makes other people think we are clumsy.

I heard the chair scrape on the floor as Mrs. Brooks pulled it out for me. Somehow, I got myself seated. The kids on each side of me asked, "What's wrong with your eyes?"

"I got lye in them," I said.

"What's lye?" they asked.

"Something your pour in the sink when it's stopped up," I managed to say. I wanted to leave.

The kid on my right said, "Oh, I am glad I don't look like you."

The kid on my left said, "Oo oo."

I heard one person clapping the way Grandmomma clapped when she wanted Billy and me to pay attention. Mrs. Brooks said, "We will now color a picture."

Someone put a piece of paper in my hands. I heard the rustle of papers being passed out to what I figured was the rest of the class. "Here are your crayons," Mrs. Brooks said and put a box in my hands.

I opened the box and smelled the crayons. I loved their smell. I held the box close to my left eye and looked for a red one.

"Children," Mrs. Brooks said, "what outline do you see on your piece of paper?"

The piece of paper looked and felt blank to me.

"A house!" everyone else shouted.

"Go ahead and color," Mrs. Brooks said.

But I couldn't see the outline. I put my face down on the piece of paper but I couldn't see an outline at all. I wondered what a house looked like. I knew the outside of some houses felt like wood and some felt like brick.

I decided to color up and down on the paper with the red crayon. I had heard of red-brick houses.

"You're not staying in the lines," the kid next to me said. "You must be blind."

"Peggy," Mrs. Brooks said quietly over my shoulder, "Why don't you just sit still while the other children finish coloring their pictures?"

Sitting still was not my thing. I was always doing something. But I just sat there and listened to the sound of the other kids coloring and wanted to cry

***

That night, as Billy and I ate roast beef and potatoes on our TV trays, I told him about my day. Billy seemed much older and wiser than I.

"Those kids were mean to you," Billy said. "You can't help it if you can't see. I'm going to beat those kids up."

Well, I thought I might just tell those kids what my big brother had said.

In 1959, no kindergarten in America had accommodations for kids with disabilities. My mother had made a very interesting decision. She told me later that she hadn't wanted me to live away from the family at a school for the blind. She also wanted me to live in the sighted world starting at an early age. Certainly, I learned to live in the sighted world, but I missed out on things by not being with other blind children. Adults I know who attended schools for the blind have remained close to their blind classmates, but I have never had a close blind friend.

***

Things got worse at kindergarten. Before long it was October, and Mrs. Brooks wanted us to cut out Halloween pumpkins—and then in November, Thanksgiving turkeys—and then in December, Christmas

Santas. I just sat and listened to the other kids opening and closing their scissors and cutting away on construction paper. After Christmas, Mrs. Brooks said, we would start practicing for a play. Some of the girls would be sunbeams and wear yellow costumes and dance across the stage at the elementary school where we would perform. I wanted to be a sunbeam, but Mrs. Brooks said I wouldn't be able to do the dancing. She said I needed to wear a blue dress and sing a song with this boy who would wear a blue seersucker jacket.

Grandmomma said the boy seemed kind of retarded. I guessed that meant he was dumb because some of the kids in the class said he was dumb. I asked Billy what "retarded" meant. He said he thought retarded people were dumb, but they couldn't help it. So, he said, you shouldn't make fun of them.

Becky, one of the girls in my kindergarten class, was chosen to be a sunbeam. She said she felt sorry for me, and that she wanted me to spend the night at her house. I was thrilled that Becky had invited me. Everyone liked her, and she had chosen me to spend the night. The only thing I didn't like was that she said she felt sorry for me.

***

Becky lived in a two-story house across the street. When we stepped inside it felt warm, not drafty like Grandmomma's house. It smelled fresh, not musty like where we lived. Before Becky guided me up the steps, she said there were fourteen of them. I counted, and she was right. Falling up steps is not too frightening, but falling down steps is the number-one fear of all blind people. Becky guided me to her room and put my hand on her bed. I immediately felt a lot of stuffed animals. I picked up a bear and gave him a big hug.

"I love animals," Becky said. "Either China or stuffed. Let me let you feel my collection of China animals."

I immediately recognized the China giraffe with his long neck and the elephant with his tusks. She let me feel a lion, a tiger, and a bear. "I keep them on my bedside table."

I listened as Becky replaced the animals one by one on her bedside table.

"What color is your room?" I asked.

"It's painted yellow," she said "I have two windows with white curtains trimmed in lace."

I usually slept in Grandmomma's little front bedroom, where some of the wallpaper was falling off the walls. Becky's bedroom had the sound of a big room to me. As we sat on Becky's bed, I told her the newest rhyme I had learned: "Milk, milk, lemonade, around the corner, fudge is made." I pointed to the appropriate body parts. Becky laughed and said she was going downstairs to ask her mother what we were going to have for dinner. She closed the door to her bedroom behind her. I heard her light footsteps run down the stairs. Carefully, I felt for the China elephant on the bedside table. My little suitcase was at the end of the bed. I placed the China elephant in the bottom of my suitcase and zipped it up. Becky ran back into the room and said she had told her brother the rhyme, and her brother told their mother and their mother slapped him. On top of that, Becky didn't have a chance to ask her mother what we were having for dinner. At that point I wanted to leave, but I was determined to spend the night. I knew that when I would have to talk to Becky's mother that night, I would feel uneasy.

In a little while there was a knock on Becky's bedroom door. "What do you want, Jimmy?" Becky asked.

"Time for supper," he said, as the door squeaked open a crack.

Becky said I might want to hold on to the rail as we walked down the staircase. And so, I did.

"Momma has the table set on this side for two," Becky said as we walked into what had to be the dining room. "Jimmy will sit across from us, and Momma at one end of the table. Daddy is out of town."

We sat down, and I heard Mrs. Smith ask, "Jimmy, please say the grace."

"'God is great, God is good. Let us thank him for our food. By His hand we all are fed. Give us Lord our daily bread.'"

"Thank you Jimmy," Mrs. Smith said. "Peggy, you have a hamburger and a bun and some French fries on your plate. Do you want some ketchup?"

I did, but I didn't want Mrs. Smith to serve me any. I was scared of her.

"No, Ma'am, but thank you," I said.

"Peggy likes the clock method," Becky said. "So, your hamburger and the bun are at three, four and five o'clock. And your French fries are at six, seven and eight."

Becky didn't seem scared of her mother. I ate as quickly as I could, remembering to close my mouth to chew.

"Peggy and I are finished," Becky said as I swallowed my last mouthful. "Mom, can we be excused?"

"You may both be excused," she said.

We made it okay through supper, but I sure hoped Becky didn't see the missing China elephant in her room.

The next morning when the doorbell rang, and I heard my grandmother's voice, I was so glad. I could now escape with the stolen elephant. I rushed home with Grandmomma and up to my little bedroom. I opened my suitcase but the back leg of the elephant had broken off. I never stole anything again.

***

The next day Momma went to the hospital. "Why did Momma go to the hospital?" I asked my grandparents.

"She's depressed," Granddaddy said.

Billy and I had pork chops with baked apples and sweet potatoes and baked onions and rice and gravy on our TV trays that night. I asked Billy again what "depressed" was.

"Remember, Piglet, it means you are sad a lot and you cry a lot," he said. "You know how Momma didn't come out of her room lately? When I saw her eyes the other day, it looked like she had been crying."

I needed to think that over. "Depressed" was a big word for a kid in kindergarten. I was scared. Would Momma come back home soon? Would I smell her Arpege perfume again? Would she ask me to run downstairs and get her purse and bring it to her in bed? That way she could pull out her cigarettes and smoke another one? Were there kids who never saw their mother again?

***

One day Grandmomma and Granddaddy took Billy and me to see Momma in the hospital. The place smelled so clean. We had to sit in a waiting room and someone brought Momma out to meet us. I heard a heavy door open and close, but just before it closed, I heard someone scream. Then Momma was hugging Billy and me. She was crying. She stopped and said, "I'll be home soon, little darlings. Granddaddy bought us a house. You will each have a nice bedroom. We will get a dog and have birthday parties, and everything will be nice."

"Can I have a piñata for my birthday party?" Billy asked.

"Yes, you can. And Peggy, you can too."

"What's a piñata?" I asked. I looked outside, and the sun was shining.

"It's an animal made of papier-mâché that you hang on a tree. You take turns hitting it with a stick, and when it breaks open, candy falls all over the ground," Billy said importantly.

"Can you come home today?" Billy asked. "We want you to come home."

"No," Momma said, but at least she had stopped crying.

"Can you come home tomorrow?" I asked.

"No," Momma said, "but I promise to come home soon. I love you with all my heart."

"Come on, children," Grandmomma said, and I could hear from the level of her voice that she was standing.

Billy and I both hugged Momma, and she hugged and kissed us. Daddy had been gone for a long time. I was so confused. I held on to Billy's arm as we walked outside. "You can see through the windows of the lobby and waiting room," Billy whispered. "But you can't see in to the windows of the hospital rooms. They are covered with something white."

Billy and I sat quietly in the back of Granddaddy's Packard. I pretended to be asleep. Grandmomma said, "Mary Jean wasn't crying as much."

"But she has to have another shock treatment," Granddaddy said.

I wondered what a shock treatment was. I would have to ask Billy later. I couldn't get a handle on all this. Daddy was gone. Momma was in the hospital. I was blind. My friend Becky could see, and she had both her parents with her.

As an adult, I learned that shock treatment was supposed to re-fire the neurons in the brain to alleviate depression. Based on my reading of *One Flew Over the Cuckoo's Nest*, I believe the treatments could still be brutal in 1960. According to author Ken Kesey, arms and legs were often broken. He depicted the atmosphere of a mental hospital as a dismal place where patients were overly drugged and had no decision-making power. I'm sure my mother was suicidal as well. Not once in my life did I hear my mother mention her shock treatments.

I think it was Momma's love for Billy and me and her religious faith that sustained her. When she could think clearly in her hospital bed, psalms and hymns and the sound of our laughter must have filled her mind.

Chapter Four

At Grandmomma's that night I was in the sitting room with Billy. I got up to pace around and ran into the piano bench. Then the coffee table. "Bad coffee table," Billy said. "Bad, bad piano bench."

I asked him about shock treatment, but he really didn't know what it meant. "I'm going outside," he said.

I knew Billy didn't like to talk about serious things too much.

I felt the sofa I was sitting on. It had two slipcovers: one for summer and one for winter. Since it was winter, I knew the sofa had on what Grandmomma had described as a dark green winter slipcover. The winter one had a smoother feel than the summer one. Grandmomma had told me that the summer slipcover was white.

If I knelt on the sofa facing backward and spread my arms wide, I could feel the books on the huge floor-to-ceiling bookcase behind the sofa. My grandfather kept all his legal books there, along with some novels. Most prized were some slightly worn family Bibles at the end of one shelf. The names William McCann Paul "Billy" and Margaret Mason Paul "Peggy," along with our birthdates, appeared in the Daniel family Bible.

I felt a large, old-fashioned radio sandwiched between the sofa and the bookcase. It was made of smooth wood. I felt the mesh front and pushed it inward. Grandmomma had told me the mesh covered the speaker. Momma said she used to listen to "Little Orphan Annie" on the radio. Grandmomma said the family used to listen to FDR's Fireside Chats on the radio until she and Granddaddy decided the country was going to the dogs and FDR was responsible.

Only at suppertime did the TV trays sit between the coffee table and the sofa. Otherwise, the coffee table stood alone. On it sat four plastic blocks, each with different-colored sides. Grandmomma called the set of blocks a conversation piece. I could only see the red sides. Billy said the other sides were blue, green, orange, yellow, and white. The idea was to put all the greens in a row, all the reds in a row, and so on. Perhaps it was a forerunner to the Rubik's Cube.

Grandmomma also had a small black-and-white TV on the coffee table. It was the one on which she watched the news and the game show "Jeopardy." Sometimes she would turn her black-and-white TV into what she called a poor man's color TV. This meant she would put a translucent, snap-on cover over the regular TV screen. Billy said the cover made the TV screen look blue at the top and green at the bottom, and that in between the blue and green were sections of yellow and red. If the picture on the TV screen was of a blue sky with a yellow sun and a red house and green grass, then everything looked fine. Otherwise, the picture looked strange. Grandmomma had a stack of *Town & Country* magazines on the coffee table as well. Sometimes I liked to pick up a print magazine and pretend I was reading it. But usually, Billy would come along and say, "You have that magazine upside down, Piglet." His nickname for me wasn't meant to be mean. It was just a play on my name, Peggy.

Sometimes our dog, Beany, thumped her tail on the sitting-room rug, and I could hear it. Other times, if Beany was sleeping quietly, I might trip right over her, and she'd growl, and I would bump into a piece of furniture. It is incredible how much time blind people spend running into things.

Against one wall stood an antique secretary. I would feel the glass doors on the front of the top cabinet, which housed books, even though I knew Clara might say something to me about my fingerprints on the glass. Below the glass was a flat, horizontal piece of wood that opened out into a desktop. It was locked with a key, which I would turn in its lock so I could pull the desktop down and feel the felt covering on its surface. Billy said the felt was green. Then I would close the desktop and secure it with the key.

Next, I would sit on the floor, making sure not to sit on Beany, and open the wooden doors at the bottom of the secretary. The bottom cabinet contained games like Parcheesi and Tiddlywinks. I liked to feel each tiddlywink, which were smooth, round, hard plastic discs the size of a dime or a nickel. I couldn't see to play the game. When I turned eight,

Grandmomma bought me a deck of Braille playing cards. We kept them in the secretary. The bottom of each card was marked in Braille with letters like AH for the ace of hearts, or 2D for the two of diamonds. I prided myself on the saying that I had a marked deck. I learned to play Go Fish and Hearts and regular Solitaire on those cards.

Grandmomma also had an upright piano in her sitting room. I could feel the framed pictures on top of the piano when I stood on the bench. Momma didn't mind if I stood on piano benches, but Grandmomma greatly minded. Billy said a lot of the pictures were of him, Momma, and me before I was blinded.

The first song I learned to play on the piano was "I Am Mr. Middle C." Sometimes Clara came in and played "East Side / West Side" or "Lawd, I Ain't No Stranger Now."

I sang with her,

"Lawd, I ain't no stranjuh now,
Lawd, I ain't no stranjuh now,
I am introduced to the Father and the Son
Lawd, I ain't no stranjuh now."

Momma came home from the hospital after six months. I had just finished kindergarten, and I had not yet entered first grade. It was the summer of 1960. Momma, Billy, and I moved into the bungalow Granddaddy bought for us. Our new house had a living room, a dining room, a kitchen, two bedrooms, and one bathroom. Billy said every room was painted pink. Momma said as soon as she could afford it, she would have every room in the house painted turquoise. A few walls were papered with ballerinas. Momma wanted to have these walls wallpapered in silver. Granddaddy had installed burglar bars on all the windows.

Regarding the two bedrooms, Momma gave one to Billy and one to me, while she slept on a daybed in the dining room. As an adult, now I realize what a sacrifice Momma made so that Billy and I could each have our privacy. She didn't have much of her own with her bed in the dining room and the two of us constantly dashing in and out.

When we visited my grandparents, Momma usually played Bach or Beethoven on the old upright. I sat next to the piano in my grandfather's easy chair and turned on the floor lamp. It had three levels and as I turned it up, I could detect the increases in light. I have always loved light. I have sometimes reached to pick up bright sunbeams off a dark floor.

Sometimes I sat on the living room sofa with my grandfather. Occasionally I turned around and felt the wooden curly-Q design on top of the upholstered back. My grandfather read to me, and I always brought my Tiny Tears doll along to listen. He read to me, and I wished my eyes looked like Tiny Tears' eyes felt. He read me Bible stories and Bobbsey Twins books. My favorite Bible story was David and Goliath, and my favorite Bobbsey Twins book was *The Bobbsey Twins and Baby May*. Every night my grandfather asked to see my fingernails and cleaned them with his pocketknife.

Momma adored her father, and she placed him on the highest pedestal as he did her. Momma had a lot of conflict with her mother. For some reason, her mother wanted her to constantly go to parties at the Yacht Club, but Momma wanted to lie in bed and read *David Copperfield* or *The Mayor of Casterbridge* or *Tess of the D'Urbervilles*.

Shortly after we moved into our house, Granddaddy died of a brain aneurysm. I remember Momma crying and crying, but she didn't go back to the hospital for her depression. I was considered too young to go to the funeral. I remember only that someone brought me a lovely stuffed dog to cheer me up.

***

Billy and I made up a game we called Get Across. We had a long, wide living room in our new house. In the game, my base was a built-in bookcase and Billy's base was the front door directly across from it. When it was my turn, I was supposed to crawl across the rug (which smelled like Beany) and touch Billy's base.

"You're first," Billy shouted. "On your mark, get set, go!"

I crawled as fast as I could to what I knew was Billy's base. He tackled me. He sat on my chest and pinned my arms to the floor. His breath smelled like a Hershey bar.

"Momma, tell Billy to get off me!" I yelled.

Momma was smoking a cigarette and reading *David Copperfield*. "Settle it yourselves," she said in a calm voice.

I offered Billy a Mickey Mantle baseball card and a piece of flat pink bubble gum. Billy said that suited him fine, and he let me go.

To this day, I find it amazing that my mother did nothing to intervene. Here sat my older, sighted brother on top of his younger, blind sister. Yet I am very grateful to my mother for allowing me to be an equal to my brother. I rejoice in it.

As an adult, Billy says the game "Get-Across" taught me resourcefulness. And I believe it did. I am good at getting myself out of jams. After all, who doesn't want a Mickey Mantle baseball card, and a piece of flat, pink bubblegum to settle a score!

"Now let's go play Imaginary Man," Billy said.

"Okay," I said.

I walked over to Momma's bed in the dining room and coughed on cigarette smoke. "Hello, darling," Momma said, "Look out for the floor lamp I pulled over here. It is usually beside the piano. Don't trip on the cord."

I tried to avoid the cord but stepped on Beany's tail. She growled.

"I'm sorry, Peggy. I'm sorry, Beany," Momma said.

"Come on," Billy yelled from the back door.

Momma said, "Give me a kiss and then run along and play."

I could smell the smoke, but Momma always moved the cigarette out of the way of kisses. I heard Beany head toward the back door. "Sooey, piggy, piggy," Billy called from the back door.

"Good-bye Momma," I said.

"I love you, Peach Cake," she replied.

Billy slammed the back door, which meant Beany had gone outside. But where?

I pushed open the back screen door and ran down the four steps. I didn't take time to pet Wicky, the cat, who was always sitting on the stair rail. The light was bright outside. At the bottom of the steps I called, "Where's Beany?"

"She ran down the alley toward the park. She'll be gone for a while."

I found the pecan tree we used as home base. Billy put a kickball in my hands. It smelled like rubber. I put it on the ground in front of me to kick. I kicked the ball and headed for the oil drum that was first base. "I have the ball," Billy yelled. "But I will let you touch first. Leave an Imaginary Man there and go back home."

As I headed for home, I sang the song "Jenny" to myself:

"Jenny made her mind up at seventy-five,
That she would live to be the oldest woman alive.
But Gin and Rum and destiny played their tricks,
And Jenny kicked the bucket at seventy-six."

I tripped over the ball. "The ball is right in front of you," Billy said.

I felt ashamed. I couldn't see the ball. But I covered it up. "Duh, now," I said.

I put out my hand and touched the pecan tree. I found the ball with my foot and kicked it forward. I headed back to first while my Imaginary Man headed to second. Second was a Crepe Myrtle tree.

I went back to home base and kicked again. Billy immediately tapped my arm with the ball. "You're out!" We played for just one out.

I walked to the pecan tree in the middle of the yard that was where the pitcher stood. "Roll the ball here, here, here," Billy called from home base.

I rolled the ball, and I heard his shoe connect with it. I heard the whoosh of the ball in the air and the sound as it landed in the neighbor's yard.

"Home run!" Billy shouted.

"I'm going inside to talk to Momma."

What did the Imaginary Man teach me other than at times I 100 percent lose? I resented the game and always felt depressed after playing it. I wished I could cry, but I never could.

Still, I had Billy on quite a pedestal, partly because he was so smart and partly because he was the only male among Grandmomma, Momma, Clara and me. He called me "Piglet" which was a sweet nickname from *Winnie the Pooh*. He also called me "lame brain idiot" sometimes, which was kind of insulting, but really made me laugh.

I was grateful that Billy exclaimed "bad chair" whenever I ran into one, and he threatened to beat up kids who made fun of my eyes.

I found Momma still reading in bed. "Don't take it too seriously," she said.

I wanted to cry out, "Why do you let Billy play Imaginary Man with me since I can't ever win?" Sometimes I hated my mother. "Momma," I burst out, "What happened to me?"

"I told you about the plumber unstopping our kitchen sink with Lye. You stood by me; I was ironing. You ran over to watch him. At just that moment he plunged the lye, and it struck you in both eyes."

I knew Momma was upset, but I didn't care. I crossed my arms. I heard Beany's collar jingle. She thumped her tail against the dining room wall, and I knew where she was. "Let's sing a song," Momma said rather quickly. "How about 'Romeo'?"

"Romeo went roamin'
That's how he won his name.
Romeo went roamin'
That's how he won his fame.
A roamin' in the gloamin'
He came upon Juliet.
With his cute little ladder
He didn't think he had her,
But he said I'll get you yet—

"But why?" I cried out.

"Suffering is a mystery," Momma said. "Anyway, being blind is better than having a bad disposition. Now go outside and play. I want to finish *David Copperfield*, even though I've read it three times."

I headed toward the front door. Beany followed me. I felt for her ears. German shepherds have the softest fuzz on their ears. Hers felt like velvet. I opened the door and stepped onto the porch. Beany rushed by me, and I heard her toenails click down the steps.

I turned left and felt for the big wooden porch swing and for the rightmost of the two chains from which the swing hung. I softly sang a nonsense song that Billy's class had learned last year.

"Chew chocolate covered mothballs
Drink Wrigley's spearmint beer.
Kennel Ration dog food makes your wife's complexion clear;
Simonize your baby with a Hershey's candy bar.
See the difference Drano makes in every movie star."

I knew Drano contained lye, but also that this was a silly song.

I swung as high as I could in the porch swing. I had to get my mind on something else. Robert Louis Stevenson occurred to me.

"How I do like to go up in a swing,
Up in the air so blue?
Oh, I do think it the pleasantest thing
ever a child can do!"

I heard kids talking and their footsteps walking by in front of my house. I didn't recognize their voices. I automatically covered my eyes with one hand. I knew I would be much prettier if I hadn't gotten lye in both my eyes.

***

Often when I was in first grade and Billy was in third grade, we played this game where we chased each other around and around a wall. It was the wall that separated our dining room from our kitchen. If I started at the dining room door that led into the hall and turned right and then turned right again immediately into the kitchen and then ran forward along the wall and turned right, I'd be back in the dining room. Billy was always right behind me. Momma never said anything.

I never ran into the wall. I had to navigate through three doorways. But why was I unafraid to run? I just didn't think I would run into the wall or the doors that were propped open. My goal was to run as fast as I could. I'm sure my brother tagged me, but I just kept running. I loved that glorious sense of running and knowing where I was. In a strange place I had to walk slowly and feel my way along.

Chapter Five

In first grade I often stood in front of the double dresser that was in my bedroom facing the mirror that hung above it. I stared as hard as I could, but I could not see myself. I could only see the light reflecting on the mirror, and I said to myself, "I would have been such a pretty girl."

I felt so bad. Why was I blind? What had happened to me? Some kid said my right eye looked white with red in it, and the other eye had a little blue. My prosthesis, when I had one, felt uncomfortable and never improved the appearance of my right eye very much. I pulled on my eyelids by the eyelashes just to have some contact with my eyes.

I thought about what my nine-year-old friend Maureen said sometimes. "You would have been a really pretty girl if you could see." Or what my eight-year-old friend Carol said to me, "Your eyes look bad, but, oh, well...."

Anytime someone wanted to take my picture, I turned my back to the camera. I did this because when other kids saw my photos they said, "Oooh, look at your eyes."

Photographers made me look their way when they took school pictures, and I wanted to throw the pictures away when I got them. However, Billy always brought home his school pictures, so Momma asked about mine as well. Even though Billy was in a different elementary school, our pictures were taken around the same time.

I spent countless hours trying to see myself in that mirror. I have never recovered from my unhappiness over the blindness and the disfigurement. It was seemingly more than I could deal with, and yet I have dealt with it.

Sometimes I thought about the witch in *Snow White*: "Mirror, mirror on the wall, who's the fairest of them all?"

As I grew older, I realized the importance of appearance in women's lives. Women constantly look in mirrors to reassure themselves that they look okay.

***

One time at the age of seven when I was in first grade, I was lying on my box spring and mattress in my bedroom. I was always relaxed in bed, because I didn't have to navigate the world. I heard Momma's high heel shoes clacking on the kitchen floor. When she got home from teaching every afternoon, she took her heels off to lie in bed and read *David Copperfield* or *The Mayor of Casterbridge*. But once in a while in the evening, she put her high heels back on to go out briefly with a girlfriend. They would just run to the drugstore for a Coke leaving Billy, Beany, and me in charge for a few minutes. Anyway, it sounded like Momma was standing now in the kitchen near the stove. I heard the sound of her taking a shoe off and then, with all her might, slamming it against the back door. I sat bolt upright in bed. What was Momma doing? I didn't think I should say anything. My room was dark, but I looked toward my door, and I could see the kitchen light was on. I crawled under my sheet and bedspread. I put my pillow over my head and put my thumb in my mouth. Then I carefully pulled the pillow away from one ear to listen. I heard Momma pick the shoe up. She must have taken the other shoe off because I heard her walk in her bare feet back through the kitchen and into the dining room.

As an adult, I have wondered why my mother acted that way that evening. I guess things just came to a breaking point.

***

Momma made sure Billy and I went to Sunday school at St. Johns Presbyterian Church. My first grade Sunday school teacher's name was Miss Whitner. Momma dropped me off early at my class the first day and left me at the altar by myself. I was never in another Sunday school class where the teacher had an altar. This one was covered in velvet, which Miss Whitner told me later was dark green. I felt a flat round bowl on the altar, and Miss Whitner said later it was an offering plate made of brass, and she had two of them. I liked Miss Whitner's voice. It sounded Southern and friendly.

A lot of light streamed into the room, so I thought it had many windows on the outside wall. I stepped away from the altar and began to feel a semicircle of small wooden chairs arranged on a thick rug. I heard the door open, and Miss Whitner said, "Hello, Peggy. I am surprised to see you here so early."

"Hello, Miss Whitner. What color are the chairs and the rug in your classroom?"

"The rug is dark green, and the chairs are tan," she said. "If you step off the rug you will be standing on a white tile floor."

I heard the door open again, and the voices of many children streamed into the room. This first Sunday, and every Sunday thereafter, we sat in the wooden chairs and sang a song. Today we sang "Noah Built Himself an Ark." Then Miss Whitner read us a Bible story about Noah, and the sighted children mentioned they could see the pictures in the book, which she held up for them. I really didn't know what a lot of animals looked like. I had recently felt a stuffed giraffe with its long neck and an elephant with its trunk and long tusks.

Next, Miss Whitner asked two children to pass the offering plates, starting at each end of the semicircle. I didn't have any money with me, but it bothered me that the child on my right passed the offering plate right over me to the child on my left. I would like to have passed the plate. I did hear some coins fall into the plate, but not that many, so I figured a lot of other kids didn't have money either. Next Miss Whitner told all the kids to go to little tables to color pictures of animals who boarded the ark. I could not color, but Miss Whitner gave me a stuffed kangaroo to play with, and I stayed in my seat in the semicircle. The stuffed kangaroo had a baby kangaroo in its pouch. I wondered if the other kids were staring at me sitting by myself. I didn't understand eyesight.

When the class ended, Miss Whitner and all the other kids left. She said she didn't want to leave me by myself, but she had to go to choir, and my mother would pick me up soon. While I waited, I thought I would like to do something fun. I felt my way to one side of the semicircle of chairs. I started with the first chair and pushed all the chairs together. Now they were in a semicircle with no space between them. I stood up on the first chair and began walking confidently around the semicircle. When my mother opened the door, she didn't say anything about my walking on the chairs. She just said, "You ready to go, Peacharoo?"

A good friend of our family told me some years later that she walked by the classroom that day and saw me through the window in the door walking around on the chairs. She was amazed. She said she didn't want to open the door because it might startle me. She said my walking around on the chairs showed my desire for independence and my daring.

***

In November of 1960, Momma took me to Delray Beach to have my false eye made. Clara rode with us and sat in the passenger seat drinking a Coca Cola. In Momma's car, Clara always sat in the passenger seat. In Grandmomma's car, she always sat in the back, regardless of whether Momma or Grandmomma was driving.

We were going to stay outside Delray with Momma's long-time friends, Ruth and Wally Bennett. Mrs. Ruth always dressed up as a witch at Halloween, which was the next day. She gave out Halloween gifts instead of candy. Clara liked the cook at the Bennett house. Her name was Dora. They had always had a good time talking in the kitchen.

As we rode along, I said, "Clara, can you tell me a story about Momma?"

"The day she was born, your grandfather took your Uncle Herbert, who was six years old, to see the baby in the hospital. I can see him right now. He had on a blue coat with a blue hood all trimmed in red. He stuffed his pockets full of toys to take to his new baby sister. A brand-new baby couldn't play with toys, but he didn't know that."

"A policeman is pulling us over," Momma said.

Momma pulled over to the side of the road. The policeman got out of his car and came to Momma's window.

"What is she drinking?" he asked.

"She's drinking a Coca-Cola," Momma said.

"Let me see the bottle."

I guess Momma handed him the bottle.

"I will just pour the Coke off and give you back the bottle," he said. I heard the Coke pour onto the pavement. "Here's the bottle, lady," he said, presumably to Momma. "You can have it."

"Why did he do that?" I asked.

"I guess because white policemen wonder what black people are drinking out of bottles," Momma said. "It's really because we live in the South. It's totally unfair."

Clara was totally silent.

***

The next day Momma took me to see the false-eye maker. My hands were shaking. I held onto Momma's left arm with my right hand as tight as I could. We walked into Mr. Brown's office. "What was the cause?" he asked.

"Lye," Momma said, and her voice shook.

I already did not like Mr. Brown. He had not even said hello to me. Grandmomma said you should always say hello to people, and say "Nice to meet you" or "Nice to see you."

"What color were her eyes?" Mr. Brown asked. He had one of those high men's voices that bothered me.

"Blue," Momma said, and she didn't sound happy. I was sitting in a leather chair with a hard back that felt way too big for me. "Put your head back," Mr. Brown said. "I'm going to put a glass conformer in."

He pushed and pulled upon my right eyelid until he got the glass conformer securely in place. His actions hurt me. He poked and prodded so much, but I was scared to say anything. He said he was surprised that the first conformer he tried fit so well over my remaining eyeball. Mr. Brown said he would paint a glass eye just like the conformer to match my other eye so I could wear it as a prosthesis or false eye.

And then began the long journey in which we tried to find someone who could make a prosthesis that matched my left eye in every way. A never-ending issue was that the right prosthetic eye always opened much wider than the left eye, in spite of tremendous advancements in the making of these prosthetics. For some years they had been carefully molded from acrylic.

Recently, my daughter Meredith was looking at some of my pictures from when I was a two-year-old. "You had beautiful eyes before you were blinded," she said.

"Let's sing a song," I said:

"In Dublin's Fair City
Where the girls are so pretty
I first laid my eyes
On sweet Molly Malone.
As she wheeled her wheel barrow
In streets broad and narrow...."

On my next morning back at school, I didn't have the chance to talk to my best friend, Jackie, until we were out on the playground. "How does my new false eye look, Jackie?" I said, just as we got out on the playground.

"Hi, Peggy," she said. "It just opens so much wider than the other one."

My heart sank. I knew it felt that way, but I had hoped it didn't look that way.

"Y'all want to play 'who's the prettiest'?" said Carol, another girl in our class.

Jackie and I joined hands with Carol in the middle.

"Who's the prettiest?" we shouted. I joined in as Carol said "Jackie is" without hesitation.

I think if I could have had either the disability or the disfigurement it might have been okay. The combination seemed overwhelming. On the other hand, I learned faster and remembered more than most of my classmates. Other kids said I was smart. Teachers said I was smart. Well, I was going to be smart. I was going to raise my hand faster and make straight As on tests. I became an overachiever by the second grade. Billy was smarter, but he didn't feel that he had to make the kind of grades I did.

***

When I was in second grade, I decided I wanted to join the Catholic Church. I was sitting on my box springs and mattress one sunny morning with my friend Maureen. We couldn't put our backs against a wall because the side of the bed was pushed up against windows. Maureen had just turned nine, and I had just turned seven. Maureen kept saying she needed to lose weight by her tenth birthday. "My mom is going to paint my bedroom spring violet for my birthday," Maureen said. "I want to look prettier for my pretty room."

"Your room needs to be painted," she continued. "The turquoise paint is peeling."

"I can't see it but I pray Momma will paint it," I said. "I don't think she paints. Some friends of hers painted the living room ceiling, though."

"Catholic prayers reach God faster," Maureen said. "That's why I'm glad I'm a Catholic."

"I want to be a Catholic," I said.

"It's the best religion," Maureen said "What do you think your mother would say if you asked to become a Catholic?"

That night Billy and I fought over whose turn it was to do the dishes. I lost and had to wash the dishes and fit them into the draining rack. Afterward, I asked Momma in the kitchen if I could become a Catholic. To my mother's great credit, since this came from a seven-year-old child, she said, "When I have an important question to ask, I ask a minister."

As an adult, I'm amazed that my mother didn't say, "We are Presbyterians, and you need to stay with your family."

I said to Momma, "Maybe I could ask Mr. Blackburn."

Mr. Blackburn served as a Methodist minister, and he and his family lived next door to my grandmother. His son Robert and Billy were friends. I was afraid of grown men. My father had been gone a long time. And of course, my grandfather had recently died. That night I got the Blackburn's number from Billy and gave Mr. Blackburn a call. His wife said he was busy but would call me back in a few minutes.

When the phone rang, I picked it up, and Mr. Blackburn said his name.

"I have a question," I said. "I'm a Presbyterian but would like to become a Catholic. My best friend is a Catholic. I was wondering if it was a good idea."

And Mr. Blackburn laughed.

I held on to the edge of the dresser where the phone sat. I didn't cry. I just didn't know what to say. I looked toward the windows, and it was dark outside.

"I think you should stay at the same church with your folks," said Mr. Blackburn, and he continued to laugh.

I didn't have folks. I just had Momma and Billy. I have never gotten over Mr. Blackburn laughing at me that way. I can hardly tell the story even today. Momma has always had an incredibly high opinion of ministers. So, I don't think it ever occurred to her a minister would laugh at the question. She thought he would take it seriously.

***

In the second grade I began to learn Braille. A Braille teacher who traveled up from St. Augustine two days a week taught Paul and me. Paul was the only other blind child in Duval County. Paul was always nice. We were bussed to the same elementary school, probably so Mrs. Williamson could teach us together. She gave us flash cards with individual words in Braille on them. We had words like "run," "go" "come," and "see." I said I sure wished I could see.

I loved Braille and learned it quickly. Soon I was reading a book about Alice and Jerry and Jip, the dog. I could finally read for myself!

Every letter and symbol in Braille is composed of a combination of just six dots; each cluster of dots, arranged in two columns of three, is called a cell. In a cell, the letter A is represented by the upper left-hand dot; B is the upper left-hand dot plus the dot underneath it; and C is the two dots going across the top.

Braille is much more complex than print because of its 300 to 400 shorthand symbols. Words like "with" and "for" are spelled out in print but are written as single-cell symbols in Braille. Also, while every letter of the alphabet is represented by a Braille character, many letters can also stand alone to symbolize a word. For example, the letter "W" standing alone is the word "will." A standalone W with one dot before it gives us the word "work;" with two dots, the word "word;" and with three dots, the word "world."

Braille books come in volumes. The volumes of the Braille Bible, stacked horizontally, stand five feet, three inches tall. When I walked into Mrs. Williamson's resource room in my elementary school, I found many bookcases containing Braille books. Even though most of them were textbooks, I liked reading them. On her supply-room door, Mrs. Williamson always posted a Braille poem. I particularly liked one called "Tain't."

Tain't what we have,
But what we give;
Tain't who we are,
But how we live;
Tain't what we do,
But how we do it—
That makes this life
Worth going through it!

While Mrs. Williamson was teaching me Braille, she also taught me how to type on both a Braille writer and a regular print typewriter. I took my Braille writer to class for some tests, like math tests, and my typewriter to class for other tests, such as spelling tests and English tests. I couldn't figure out which machine made more noise. Anyway, they both made more noise than the sound of a pencil. When Mrs. Williamson came up to the school, she transcribed the Math answers for my regular classroom teacher.

***

In second grade, at age eight, I received a D on my report card in handwriting. My friend Jacky read me my report card, and I knew my grandmother would be mad that I received all A's and a D. Momma would not be upset. But Grandmomma paid Billy and me a nickel for every A we made and certainly nothing for a B, C, or D. I couldn't write by hand very well because I couldn't see.

I knew Grandmomma would be at our house when I arrived home on the school bus. Billy walked to a different school, and I was bussed to the one school in the county that had two blind students including me. I counted five steps up to our front porch. Momma never put a hand rail there. "How's your report card?" Grandmomma asked.

She must have been standing inside the open front door. Grandmomma never hugged me, but Momma did. I wished it were a cold day so I could be taking off a coat while I talked to Grandmomma.

"I got five A's and a D," I blurted out, and I held out the report card in its sleeve in Grandmomma's direction.

"A D! In what?" she exclaimed.

"Handwriting." I was afraid she would be mad but she said, "But you can't see. I'm going to talk to the principal! Come on inside, and I'll give you a quarter for those five 'A's."

I heard Grandmomma's keys jangle as she picked them up from the round table next to our front door. "I need to put my keys in my pocketbook. I left it on the piano bench."

Grandmomma gave me a quarter, and I wondered what to do with all that money.

The next day Jacky and I were walking out to recess and Grandmomma startled me by saying "hello" in the school hallway. I guessed she had come to see the principal about my handwriting grade. My grandmother had my report card and I had to fib to my teacher this morning that my mother had not had time to sign the back of it.

That afternoon while other kids were coloring, Mrs. Lankford, the teacher, asked me to come out into the hallway with her. "I changed your handwriting grade from a D to a B," she said kindly.

As an adult, I understood Mrs. Lankford did not understand my situation. Even though I was learning Braille twice a week from a Braille teacher, Mrs. Lankford expected me to handwrite in print until my grandmother complained.

***

During second grade on a cool fall afternoon, Momma was vacuuming the living room rug. A friend of hers named Jane was bringing over some Swedish ivy she had planted in a pot. Jane was just an easygoing friend, so I didn't understand why Momma was vacuuming for Jane's visit. I walked carefully over to where I knew the wing-backed chair was beside the secretary and sat down. Grandmomma had told me this chair was covered in a dark green material with a print. Momma switched off the vacuum cleaner. Her familiar footsteps walked over to what I knew was a light gray sofa. Her rubber-soled shoes squeaked a little on the wooden floor. The doorbell rang. Beany, the dog, was in the backyard so she didn't start barking. I jumped up and ran toward the door and fell over the vacuum cleaner. I caught myself before I hit the rug. "I'm so sorry, darling," Momma said. She rushed over to me and put her hands on me. I didn't want her to touch me, because I was angry.

My leg really hurt. Why didn't Momma put the vacuum cleaner out of the way? "I have to answer the door," she said.

I made my way back to the wing-backed chair with my leg hurting when Momma showed Jane in who greeted me. Grandmomma said you should always stand when an adult entered the room, but I didn't have the strength. "Hello," I said as cheerfully as possible.

"The Swedish ivy is beautiful," Momma said, and I heard her roll the vacuum cleaner into a corner. She didn't say anything to Jane about my falling over it.

After Jane left, I didn't tell Mother my leg still hurt. She would not have liked that. As an adult, I concluded that my mother often didn't see consequences. She didn't really look ahead. By personality or habit, she was careless. How could my mother not think about the fact that I could easily fall over a vacuum cleaner sitting in the middle of the floor. Also, I had the embarrassment of someone seeing me do it.

***

By the end of second grade, I had started walking across a pipe that spanned Willow Branch Creek. It was a big round pipe with narrow ledges that my feet fit on either side. I could reach up and touch the bottom of the wooden bridge that ran above and to the right of the pipe. I walked down the grassy hill to the creek, mounted either side of the pipe, put up my right hand to touch the bottom of the wooden bridge, and sallied forth. I usually sang "Hard-hearted Hannah" as I walked along.

"Hard-hearted Hannah,
The vamp of Savannah,
The meanest gal in town…"

I was probably fifteen feet above the water in the creek. The creek was about twenty feet wide. Again, nobody ever said anything about it. I wondered why I felt like I could do anything.

Here I believe my mother's allowing me freedom helped me overcome my blindness. Surely a few adults saw me walking across that pipe and mentioned it to my mother..

***

At Grandmomma's I liked to go in the kitchen and talk to Clara. She had a rather booming voice. I asked Billy one time what she looked like, and he said she was tall and sort of big. He said she was very black.

Clara always sat me on her five-cornered wooden stool. I tried to tip it to the front or the back or the right or the left, but it was so heavy it wouldn't move.

"For dinner we're havin' fried chicken, rice and gravy, squash, string beans, lettuce-and-tomato salad with homemade mayonnaise, and hot biscuits all buttered. And iced tea. Don't that sound good?"

"It sure does," I said. I remembered Billy said Clara always wore a blue uniform with a white pinafore apron at work. He also told me that when Clara swept the front porch, she wore a newspaper hat.

"Do you think I'm pretty?"

"Of course, you're pretty. All that blonde hair."

"But my eyes."

"You can't help it, darling. God is able."

Obviously, Clara dealt with life's difficulties by believing in the power of God. As an adult, this strikes me as a good solution. As a child, I found the comment "God is able" frustrating.

Clara turned on the water at the freestanding porcelain sink. I heard it spatter on the newspaper that I knew was spread on the floor in front of the sink. "Listen, darling, I just swept this kitchen. My wig makes me hot." It was always hot in that kitchen even after Grandmomma added the air conditioner. Clara was forever cooking on the gas stove. I didn't know why at this late date Grandmomma had put an air conditioner in the kitchen. Could it be because Clara was a maid? Grandmomma had had air conditioners in the den and the front bedroom and her bedroom for as long as I could remember. I put my hand on the kitchen table next to me. I felt boxes that I knew contained cereal and crackers. I heard a dog bark in the distance.

"How is Brownie Jr.?" I asked.

"Fine. When I get home he stares at me. He has all that shiny brown fur. I always leave him plenty of water. But he's too lazy to drink it all." Clara laughed her hearty laugh. "Darlin', your Grandmomma doesn't like hearing about Brownie, Jr. She likes Beany."

"She hates Uncle Herbert's dog, Miss Muffett. When is he coming to town with that French poodle, Clara?"

"I don't know. Now, go tell your grandmother I'm ready to serve dinner."

I jumped off the wooden stool and said, "I love you, Clara."

"I love you too, precious," Clara said, and she grabbed me in a bear hug.

Clara seemed tall and large but not fat. When she engulfed me in a hug, I felt so loved.

Chapter Six

Momma's old Rambler wouldn't start one day so she got another, used Rambler. This one, she said, was blue. Sometimes she took Beany and me out for a ride. Beany hung her head out the back window. If she saw someone outside, she barked ferociously. I sat in front with Momma. We didn't have seatbelts in those days, and every time she turned left my door would fly open, and Momma would throw her right arm protectively across me. I wondered if I was just going to fall out of the car. No one seemed worried about Momma driving. As an adult, I realized the shock treatment must have worked.

One day we were riding along and Momma said she was very discouraged.

"What does that mean Momma?" I asked.

"It means I feel sad. But my father always said it isn't what happens to you, but the way you take it."

I wasn't quite sure what to think of that.

***

Almost every night, Momma, Billy and I had supper at our house in the dining room. Momma cooked things like Chef Boyardee spaghetti or split-pea soup with cut up hot dogs in it. One time I asked her why we didn't have the hot dogs separate from the soup. She said because that would be another damn pot to wash. I didn't like it when Momma said "damn." And besides, Billy and I were the ones who did the dishes.

One night I heard a match being struck, and then Momma said she was lighting two candles in the middle of the table. Momma set Swanson's turkey TV dinners on her beautiful Spode bird plates. Grandmomma had told Momma that she shouldn't use her beautiful Spode China on an everyday basis with children. Each bird plate had a different bird in the center, and the names appeared on the back of the plates. Tonight, Momma said I had the Lazuli Bunting, and Billy had the Arkansas Kingbird.

Momma always began Grace the same way. First, she said, "Bow your heads." Then she said, "Oh Lord, make us grateful for these and all thy blessings, for Christ's sake, amen."

We didn't talk much at dinner. Instead, we always wanted to play games like Animal, Vegetable, and Mineral or Ghost, and Hum, and Guess 'Em.

Tonight, I said, "Let's play Famous Initials."

"Okay," Momma and Billy said in unison.

I said, "I want to go first."

"Okay," they said.

I said, "O.G."

"Piglet, you don't know what you're talking about," Billy said.

"Oh, yes I do," I said.

Beany walked into the room and thumped her tail on the wall. Momma had told me she'd had silver wallpaper put up in that room. When we moved in, the room had pink ballerina wallpaper.

Momma and Billy were silent. Usually, I gave them initials like G.W. for George Washington.

The turkey dinner didn't taste good. I couldn't cut it up with Momma's wedding silver anyway. Momma had not cut up my food in a long time. I tried the somewhat-frozen mashed potatoes.

"Chew with your mouth closed, Piglet," Billy said.

Beany dropped on the floor, and her collar jingled. I wanted to remember where she was so I wouldn't step on her.

"Ha-ha-ha-haaaa, ha," I said to Billy, trying to imitate Woody Woodpecker.

"Otto Goldschmidt," I said.

"Who is Otto Goldschmidt?" they asked.

"The husband of Jenny Lind, the famous Swedish singer," I said.

"Oh, yes," Momma said. "The Swedish Nightingale. How do you know about her and him?"

"I'm reading a biography on talking-book records," I said.

At the time, I received many books on vinyl records that were sent out for the blind. "Well, Billy and I lose," Momma said.

"Can we turn on the air conditioner?" Billy asked.

"Yes," Momma said.

"Since you're sitting so close to it, go ahead and turn it on, Piglet."

I turned it on. The cool air came out. It felt great.

***

One night I was snuggled by myself into my king-sized bed. It had been my parents' bed. Momma said the spread was gold satin. In the middle of the spread her initials were embroidered: "MPJ." I liked to trace the fancy letters with my finger.

I remembered Daddy lying on his back on the bed when we lived in Texas. I'd crawl onto his stomach and straddle him. He would grab my feet with his hands, and I would plant one foot firmly in each of his hands. He would push me high into the air, and I loved balancing above him. I was blind, but I had no problem balancing.

I loved Daddy, and I missed him. However, since the divorce, he hardly ever called Billy and me. I felt embarrassed when kids asked me where my daddy was. I said he left home very early in the morning and came back late at night, so that was why other kids never saw him. Once in a while, Daddy said he was coming to see Billy and me in Jacksonville, but he only came one time. I asked Momma about him, and she said he drank a lot and was sort of tricky and often angry.

"Can you tell me a story about him?" I asked, somewhat fearfully.

"Well, one time when he was a roustabout in Wyoming in 1950, we were driving through the countryside. I asked if he thought there were any buffalo around,"

He said, "Absolutely not."

"Just then about a hundred buffalo thundered by. I stared straight ahead. I knew if I said anything, he might blow up at me."

***

It was hot in my room much of the year. The air conditioner only cooled the dining room and living room. Occasionally Momma turned on the attic fan which blew some air through the open bedroom windows, but it made so much noise.

At times I felt like crawling out of my bedroom window just for fun. But Granddaddy had burglar bars installed on all the windows of our house before he died. Snuggled in the bed, I was reading my *American Girl* magazine in Braille under the covers. At that moment I heard the door from the dining room into the hall open and close quickly. I heard my mother's footsteps come toward my room. I paused in reading my Braille. "Sweet dreams, darling," Momma whispered. I pretended to be asleep. I heard my mother's footsteps walk toward my brother's door.

"Billy, you need to turn off that flashlight, stop reading, and go to sleep."

"Yes, ma'am," Billy said. I heard the click of the flashlight. That was one time where being sighted was not a plus. I could read under the covers in the dark.

"Good night, Billy darling," Momma said.

I started reading again, *Ha-ha-ha-haaaa, ha,* I said to myself. I knew Momma was getting in her bed in the dining room, and that she was reading *The Mayor of Casterbridge*.

***

One morning when I was in third grade, I got up and put on a brand-new dress my uncle had given me. It was a cold day, and the dress felt like cotton. But I guess we wore cotton in Florida all year round. Momma had told me the dress was dark blue with a lighter blue pinafore. I felt the two parts of the dress, and the pinafore was a little shorter than the basic dress.

The house seemed quiet, and I wondered where Billy and Beany were. Then I remembered Billy must be out on his paper route with Beany running behind his bike. Then I heard the water running in the bathroom basin and knew Momma was in there. I had an idea. Stepping quietly in my penny loafers, I walked across the wooden floor of my room and made my way onto the linoleum floor of the kitchen. I wanted to warm up my dress. I felt for the knob on the kitchen stove that controlled the right front burner. I turned the knob to high. I placed the dress with the pinafore on top of the burner. Immediately I saw flames and smelled burning clothing. I backed away from the burner holding the skirt and pinafore out away from my legs. Momma ran out of the bathroom and smothered the flames with what I learned later was a towel. Momma asked me if I was all right but didn't say too much more about it. When I felt my dress, both the skirt and pinafore had a huge hole with ragged edges. The material smelled so burned. Taking the dress off, I put on my pajamas and carried the dress to the kitchen trashcan and threw it out. Momma said I still had to go to school, so I found another dress to wear.

Momma never criticized me for putting my dress over the burner. I'm sure she knew I learned from this mistake. I really thought my uncle would buy me another dress, but maybe Momma never told him about it.

***

I often spent the night with my grandmother when I was in third grade. After supper one night we were in the sitting room. "You need a new false eye," my grandmother said. "That one doesn't look natural. Mr. Brown didn't do a good job on it at all. And your mother just doesn't notice these things."

I hung my head. "Momma said she might take me to a different false-eye maker in a few years in Baltimore," I said, speaking in the direction of the floor.

"Well, that's too long, but I hope they can do something. 'A handicapped man can marry because a woman will marry anything, but a handicapped woman....'"

As a child, I didn't know what that meant. Anyway, Grandmomma said the handicapped, the Blacks, the Jews, and the foreigners just didn't fit in.

I wanted to leave the room but couldn't. I checked my Braille watch and realized it was time for "Jeopardy."

"Can you watch 'Jeopardy?'" I asked, and I heard her switch on the TV. So, she watched, and I listened. I was only in the third grade and didn't know any of the answers, but I loved learning. When the first commercial came on, I sang along:

"Winston tastes good like a cigarette should,
Winston tastes good like a [clap! clap!] cigarette should!"

The next morning, I walked into the sitting room, and Beany was thumping her tail on the Oriental rug. "Who's the sweetest dog?" my grandmother asked.

I faintly smelled her Vicks VapoRub. I opened the swinging door into the breakfast room so I wouldn't have to talk to her. I grabbed a piece of Dentyne chewing gum off the corner cabinet in the breakfast room and called, "Good morning, Clara," into the kitchen.

"Good morning, darling," Clara said and hugged me. I felt the starched bow tied in back of her uniform.

"What's for breakfast?"

"Scrambled eggs and bacon, and toast with marmalade, and orange juice, too."

"Can I sit in here and eat breakfast with you?"

"You can sit in here for a minute, but you need to sit in the dining room and eat breakfast with your grandmother. Servants eat in the kitchen."

"But why?" I asked.

"Just do," Clara said.

I liked to talk to Clara a lot more than I liked to talk to my grandmother. Grandmother's prejudices bothered me.

"You can sit on my stool for a minute," Clara said, and she placed my hand on one of the five corners.

"Have you heard Grandmomma say a handicapped man can marry because a woman will marry anything, but a handicapped woman?"

"You will land a man. Look at that blonde hair. You are pretty now. You was an ugly baby. All bald-headed."

This seemed strange to me because when I was a baby I could see. "But my eyes...."

"God is able," Clara said, as she did in response to any comment I made about my eyes.

I heard the door open from the breakfast room into the dining room. Grandmomma called, "Is breakfast ready? I have got to be at the beauty parlor in forty-five minutes."

"Yessum," Clara said. "I am serving it now.'

***

I heard something shatter on the hardwood floor. "Beany, stop wagging your tail and knocking ornaments off the Christmas tree!"

If the ornament had fallen on the Oriental rug, I would have heard it bounce. A blind person interprets their environment by differentiating sounds. A quarter makes a louder sound when dropped than a dime. I found one end of a string of lights and felt for the first light on the string. I held the string, firmly placing the first light between my hands. I studied it closely. I could see a bright white light, so I knew this light worked. The next light shone red so I knew it worked. The next light was dark so I knew it had burnt out.

Grandmomma had given me a rectangular box, which she said was made of brass. She said the box was filled with bulbs. I replaced the dark bulb and saw a bright light in its place. I loved testing Christmas lights. It was something I could do by myself. Nobody had to help me. This year, for the first time, Grandmomma was letting me plug and unplug the strings by myself. I finished testing four strings of lights and put them in a pile. I hoped Billy would have trouble untangling them when he put the strings on the tree. Since my brother gave me a hard time, I had to give him a hard time when I could. I smelled evergreen as it filled the room. I stood and carefully touched a branch of the tree. I pulled out a single needle and put the tiny piece in my mouth to chew. The taste of evergreen refreshed me.

This hallway had so many entrances and exits. For example, a door that led in and out of the porch; a door that led from the living room into the hall and back into the living room, and a flight of stairs going up and coming down. I walked through the door leading into the sitting room and heard my grandmother's pen as she wrote on a card. I knew she was sitting at a card table. "I want to finish these goddamn Christmas cards," she said. "I only have a few more local ones to write out."

Merry Christmas, I thought, and shrugged. Christmas for us was awful. Grandmomma was angry. Momma was depressed. Billy and I got very few Christmas presents and never fabulous surprises. I was always unhappy.

Beany's collar jingled as she shook her head and walked into the sitting room. "Who's the sweetest dog?" Grandmomma crooned.

"She just knocked an ornament off the Christmas tree and broke it!" I exclaimed.

"But she's the sweetest dog," Grandmomma said. "And, Peggy, tell Clara to sweep up the ornament pieces."

"Clara is fixing dinner, Grandmomma."

"Well, tell her I said to do it right now. The Blacks, as they insist on being called..." Grandmomma said in exasperation.

I walked right into the antique secretary trying to find the swinging door into the breakfast room and on to the kitchen.

"Peggy, for God's sake, be careful. And when are you going to get a new false eye? That one just doesn't look natural," Grandmomma continued.

I quickly pushed open the door into the breakfast room and heard it swing closed behind me. I smelled the chicken frying in the kitchen. Every time I came through the breakfast room I grabbed a piece of Dentyne chewing gum at the top of the cabinet. Clara was banging pots and pans, and water was spraying out from the faucet of the old-fashioned porcelain sink. I heard the water land on the newspaper on the floor in front of it.

"Hello, darlin'," Clara said and engulfed me in a big hug.

"You got on the blue uniform and white apron?" I asked.

"Yes, precious," Clara said. "I only wear a newspaper hat when I sweep the front porch. It keeps dust out of my wig."

"What's for Christmas Eve dinner besides fried chicken?"

"I got rice and gravy, string beans, and squash, and hot biscuits all buttered. I got lettuce-and-tomato salad and homemade mayonnaise."

To this day, no one can compete with Clara's cooking. Of course, at that time she threw bacon grease into the squash and string beans, and used Crisco to fry the chicken.

One thing Momma and I loved was Clara's homemade mayonnaise. You take one large egg, at room temperature, and a pint of Wesson oil and squeeze in a lemon, and whip it together and mayonnaise is born.

"What's for dessert?" I asked.

"I fixed the chocolate wafers with whipped cream, darlin'. Is your mother going to take me home tonight?"

"I think so. Listen, I hope I get something nice for Christmas."

"Well, God is able."

"But, Clara, I haven't gotten anything nice for the last two Christmases. The Christmas just before Granddaddy died I got my Patty Play Pal doll, and Billy got his Schwinn bicycle."

"I liked your Granddaddy. He loved me. He knew Mr. Finasee, a cotton man in Augusta, Georgia. My daddy knew Mr. Finasee. Anyway, your grandfather told your great-grandmother not to bother me. I made your uncle mind. And she didn't like that. She wanted to spoil him 'cause he was the first grandchild. Your great-grandmother was the meanest white woman I ever knew. Listen, darlin', my wig is hot, and I am ugly."

"I'm the ugly one, Clara. Look at my eyes," I said.

"You can't help it, darlin'. God is able. You'll land a man."

Sometimes I asked Clara about her marriage to Willy. She'd say, "I was married to Willy for twenty-two years, and he wasn't much. You know, you can't brag on men."

I've always wanted to write a short story called "You Can't Brag on Men." I would write it about my father, who ended up with four wives, and his father, my grandfather Paul, who left his family when the stock market crashed in 1929.

"Anyway, I'm ugly." Clara laughed.

"Momma thinks everybody looks fine," I said. "For Christmas, I wish I'd get some good presents wrapped in shiny paper with lovely dresses inside the boxes."

"I'd give you some if I could," Clara said.

"Oh, by the way, Grandmomma wanted you to sweep up the pieces of an ornament Beany knocked on the floor off the tree."

I heard Grandmomma's short steps coming through the breakfast room toward the kitchen. "Clara, have you seen the bowl and sponge I use to wet the postage stamps?" Grandmomma asked.

"No'm," Clara said.

"Well, I told Peggy to tell you to sweep up the ornament pieces that the sweetest dog accidentally knocked off the Christmas tree."

"I was just starting to tell her when you came in," I said.

"All right," Grandmomma said and stomped out of the kitchen.

Grandmomma seemed so angry about everything except when she was talking to her high-society friends. Then she was usually polite. Occasionally she got mad at one of these friends and referred to her as a snake in the grass. At that point she would say, "Eunice and I" or "Charlotte and I" or "Marian and I do not speak."

"Anyway, darlin', the reason your grandmother is mad is that Miz Buchanan forgot to pick her up for a debut party at the Yacht Club yesterday." Clara was referring to Grandmomma's neighbor, Alice Buchanan. "Your grandmother was ready, 'cept she needed Miz Buchanan to come zip her up before they went to the party. Miz Buchanan called today and said she forgot to call your grandmother yesterday to say that her dog Katinka got sick, and she couldn't go to the party. So now your grandmother doesn't want anything to do with Miz Buchanan."

My grandmother had told me many times how she'd broken her right arm as a child of three, and the doctors couldn't set it correctly. Since then, she'd had limited use of it and couldn't zip up her dresses.

"Your grandmother said she would have taken L.P. and driven to the party, but she wasn't zipped."

"I understand," I said. "L.P." stood for Lover Poo. He was a blow-up half-man dressed in a coat and tie. Grandmomma sat him in the passenger's seat when she was alone in the car. She thought he looked like a real man from a distance.

"When Miz Buchanan called earlier to apologize about yesterday, she said she would drive down the alleyway with some presents. She's pulling up now."

Clara bustled out of the back door onto the back porch, and I heard the screen door slam. As far as Christmas presents from Mrs. Buchanan went, she would give Beany a can of flea powder from her dog Katinka, and she would usually give Billy and me soap-on-a-rope. The soap would probably be in a shape of a dog, since she was so crazy about Katinka. I could always tell by its scent that the soap was Ivory.

Clara must have turned off the chicken, because I couldn't hear it frying anymore. I liked white meat, and I couldn't wait to get those slightly peppery morsels in my mouth.

I knew Grandmomma had a gas stove, because anytime we had a hurricane, and the electricity went out at Momma's house, we could go over to Grandmomma's to eat hot food. Just then, the doorbell rang. I walked carefully through the breakfast room and over to the swinging door into the sitting room. I opened the door and said, "Grandmomma, Clara can't answer the front door because she has gone out to the alley to get the presents from Mrs. Buchanan."

"All right," Grandmomma said. "It's probably Mrs. Elliott."

Then I remembered that Grandmomma had said Mrs. Elliott was coming with her Christmas presents today. She always gave Billy and me our nicest Christmas presents, and she always brought sour-cream cake and brownies. Mrs. Elliott's husband and my grandfather had been law partners together.

I closed the door, walked over, and felt the table in the breakfast room. The wood was rough in places and smooth in others. The table had been burned in the Jacksonville fire of 1901. A man had started the fire by throwing a lighted cigarette onto a mattress in a mattress factory. My grandmother was four, and her family had just moved to Jacksonville from St. Simons Island, Georgia. Her father sent a telegram back home that read, "Jacksonville burning up, everything fine."

Clara bustled in through the back door. "Miz Buchanan says Merry Christmas, and she gave us a whole bag of presents."

I heard the paper bag crinkling, then I heard Grandmomma's short quick steps coming into the kitchen. "Clara, here's a plate of sour-cream cake and brownies that Mrs. Elliott brought." She set the plate down. "Is that a bag of presents from Alice Buchanan?"

"Yessum," Clara said.

"Well, she probably gave me a bag of Russell Stover creams. I loathe and despise creams. But their nuts are wonderful."

I liked to stick my finger in the bottom of every Russell Stover cream to see if I could find a firm one, which generally was a caramel. Momma and I both loved chocolate. Sometimes Momma would bring home bars of Hershey's chocolate after school. I needed to find Momma. She was probably lying down.

"It's five-thirty, Clara. I would like to have dinner at a quarter of six," Grandmomma said. As an adult, I have reflected on the concept of punctuality. My grandmother was exacting about time. If she said she wanted to have dinner at a quarter to six, Clara had better have it on the table at a quarter to six. And Billy, Mother, and I had better be seated in the dining room at that very minute.

I have noticed that many people are more flexible about time. They say things like, *"Let's meet for dinner around six."* If you are five minutes late or ten minutes late, they don't care. My mother was somewhat like my grandmother about time, so I've always been time-oriented. I'm always checking to see what time it is.

"Your mother and Billy are reading on the front porch," my grandmother said. "Tell them to come in and wash their hands. And don't scream for them. Put on a sweater; I'm cold."

I hadn't brought a sweater. It seemed warm outside to me. I walked through the breakfast room and the dining room and across the Oriental rug in the hall. I felt for the smooth brass handle in the middle of the front door and opened it. I heard cars whizzing by on Riverside Avenue.

"Momma, Billy, it's time for dinner."

"After dinner, I want to play football with David," Billy said.

I headed for the powder room to wash and dry my hands. When I came out, I heard Momma and Billy talking in the sitting room near the powder-room door. I said, "I have to get by you to go into the dining room. I don't want to run into you all."

Billy grabbed me and pulled me through the sitting room to the dining-room door. Sometimes it struck me how tedious blindness was. If I could see well, I would've walked quickly out of the powder room. I would've walked right through the sitting room and into the dining room without hesitation.

When I found the dining-room table I felt for my lightweight, antique wooden chair with its woven cane seat. For fun, I stuck my fingers through the holes. I felt the linen tablecloth and what I knew was the silver napkin ring, and then put the napkin in my lap. All I could see was the blur of candle light in the middle of the table. I had felt the candelabrum when the candles were not lighted. Each candle had a bowl of glass at its base, called a "bobeche." The bobeche was designed to catch the dripping wax. "Can you say the blessing, Mary Jean?"

"Oh, Lord, make us grateful for these and all thy blessings, for Christ's sake, Amen."

In the Freedom of Space

People always said Momma was beautiful. Sometimes I was jealous.

Grandmomma was ringing the bell. "For forty years I have asked Clara to put iced tea and water at my place and for forty years she has put iced tea only."

The door from the breakfast room opened. "Can I have a glass of ice water, Clara?" Grandmomma asked with an edge to her voice.

"Yessum." I heard Clara step back and close the door from the dining room to the breakfast room. I didn't realize it as a child but as an adult I think Clara was being passive-aggressive with the ice water.

"Well, it's the second Christmas without your father, Mary Jean. His senior partner, John Smith, gave me five hundred dollars a month for only one year after your father died. He goes to church every Sunday. Damn his soul. And your father did so much free legal work for the church. God ought to do more for me, but God is powerful peculiar."

"Mother, I wish you wouldn't talk about Daddy that way." Momma, like her father, had always been a deeply religious person. She read the Bible for one hour every morning when she woke up. Even though Grandmomma didn't like Granddaddy's doing free legal work for the church, she loved his high status among the congregation.

"Let's play Ghost," Billy said, "even though there's no competition."

We played this game often, and I knew how to spell a lot of big words. The object was to make sure you weren't the one to complete the word. Two-letter words didn't count.

"S," Billy said.

"U," Grandmomma said.

"R," I said, hoping they would spell the word "Survival."

"V," Momma said.

"I," Billy said.

"V," Grandmomma said.

"A," I said.

"L," Momma said.

Momma was a third of a ghost.

"This is the best food I've ever tasted," Grandmomma said. "It's a Lucullan feast."

I knew the Roman consul Lucullus had held banquets. Favor with the host was indicated by whether you were seated above or below the salt—that is, on the side of the saltcellar near the host (above), or on the opposite side (below).

"Your turn to start a word, Piglet," Billy said.

I thought I would start with the letter "J."

"Mary Jean, I don't see why you have to wear blue jeans for Christmas Eve dinner. And you need to have your hair done."

"Johnny Terry was so bad in music class," Momma responded. Lately she had been teaching music in the junior high school. Johnny Terry's mother, Gertrude, and another friend, Martha, had come to paint our living-room ceiling a year ago. Momma said they painted it white, because it was hot pink, and Momma hated having a living-room ceiling that was hot pink.

"Don't do anything to Johnny Terry. Now you're out of school for the Christmas holidays, I need to make you an appointment with the beauty parlor. I have to go all the time. My hair is the bane of my existence."

I don't think Momma cared how her hair looked back then, but as I was growing up she got her hair done all the time. When I talk to her on the phone today she still always says she doesn't like how her hair looks. I think my grandmother gave her a complex about it.

"I don't know if I have time to go to the beauty parlor, Mother. I have to do things around my house. I have to scrub the kitchen floor with BAB-O. I have to spray for roaches. I wish I had a maid. Gertrude and Martha and all my other friends have maids."

As a child, I didn't understand why my grandmother was so mean to my mother. As I got older, I could see my mother hadn't turned out the way my grandmother wanted. I saw my Grandmomma had wished Momma would marry into a prominent Jacksonville family and live in a beautiful house on the St. John's River, and spend her days doing Junior League work. Alas, Momma had resigned twice from the Junior League. Both times because she didn't have the kind of income that the other Junior League ladies had. Momma wanted to lie in bed and read and smoke cigarettes.

"Mary Jean, I found the perfect Christmas present for myself. It's a flower-covered toilet seat. The governor of Florida's wife is ordering some for the governor's mansion. Oh, and I'll pay for the Orkin man to come spray your house once a month for roaches as a Christmas present. Now sit up straight.

"Peggy, use your biscuit to push with. Not your fingers. Manners will get you through a powerful lot of situations."

"I am as full as a tick," Billy said.

"Billy, I have told you over and over not to say you are full—certainly not to say you are as full as a tick. Say I have had a sufficiency. Or I have had a gracious plenty."

"I have had a sufficiency," I said. "Any more would be painfully superfluous." My aunt had taught me that saying.

Clara came in. "How is everything?"

"Just delicious," Momma said. "Is there any chance, Mrs. Lewis, I could have a cup of coffee?" Momma often called Clara "Mrs. Lewis."

"You certainly can have a cup of coffee, Mrs. Paul. And you, Miz Lamson?"

"No, thank you, Clara," she said in her high-toned way.

"By the way, Clara, did you sweep up the ornament?" Grandmomma asked. But Clara had left the room.

"What is the matter with you, Mary Jean?"

"I guess I'm depressed, Mother."

"Well, I'm mad," Grandmomma said. Grandmomma was more often mad, and Momma was more often depressed.

"The people who are moving into the house on the corner next door to me are pure-T common. Their son is retarded. I just don't know what that big retarded boy might do."

"In the tradition of Christmas Eve," Billy said, "can I get one present for me and one for Peggy to open?"

"All right," Grandmomma said.

Billy pushed back his chair. It was like mine, an antique with a lightweight cane bottom. I stared at the blur of candlelight and heard Billy walk quickly into the hall.

"Get the ones from the Elliotts," I called. Last year the Elliotts had given me a bright red dress. I wore it twice a week until spring, when it got too hot to wear a long-sleeved dress.

"Put out your hand, Piglet," Billy said. He put the present into my hand. I felt the satiny paper and saw it was a shiny red. I gently removed one piece of tape at a time. My grandmother saved used wrapping paper, so we had to unwrap each package carefully. Mrs. Elliott had taped each end of the box in a triangle that I could feel. I felt the lid of the cardboard box, lifted it, and felt tissue paper inside.

"A Barbie doll!" I yelled. I held her up and saw her red clothes. I felt the red velvet of the hat and coat.

Billy got a Gant shirt. "I'm going over to David's to play football," he said.

"Well, for God's sake, put on a sweatshirt," Grandmomma said. But Billy had already closed the front door behind him.

"Mary Jean, I need you to take Clara home." Ever since Grandmomma had her cataract surgery some years ago, she couldn't drive after dark. "L.P. can sit in the front seat so it looks like you have a man with you."

Clara would never sit in the front seat of Grandmomma's car. "I love Clara," Momma said, "and of course I'll take her home. I'm just tired and depressed."

"May I be excused, Grandmomma?" I asked.

"Yes," she said.

I found my way to the floor furnace between the dining room and the living room. The floor furnace was the only source of heat in that big old house. Grandmomma kept the thermostats at high in the winter so the furnace would stay on even though it didn't do much good. I thought I would go upstairs and read my Braille magazine.

"Mary Jean, would you snuff out the candles?"

"All right," Momma groused. "But then I'm taking Clara home, Mother, and coming back and going to bed."

I thought about the candle snuffer. The object was to open it up and close it over each candle flame.

"You need to comb your hair, Mary Jean."

"Mother, lay off me." Momma's steps crossed through the dining room. She opened the door of the downstairs powder room.

"I don't think Momma feels well," I said as the air from the floor furnace puffed out my dress and warmed my legs. I was standing over the furnace now.

"Oh, for God's sake," Grandmomma said. "Your mother was the girl who had the curl right in the middle of her forehead, and when she was good she was very, very good, and when she was bad she was horrid."

I felt terrible. Momma was so much nicer than Grandmomma. A few weeks ago, Momma took Billy and me to the dentist to have our teeth cleaned. We had no cavities. So, she took us to the soda fountain and we each got a hot fudge sundae.

"Your mother didn't even snuff out the candles," Grandmomma said.

I heard the powder-room door open, and Momma walked back into the sitting room. At the same time, I heard the door from the breakfast room open into the dining room and Clara said, "You want me to clear the plates, Miz Lamson?"

"Yes, I was just about to ring the bell for you."

The piano bench scraped across the Oriental rug in the sitting room. Momma began to play *"O Little Town of Bethlehem."* As Clara stacked the dishes, she joined Momma in singing:

> O little town of Bethlehem,
> How still we see thee lie;
> Above thy deep and dreamless sleep
> The silent stars go by:
> Yet, in the dark street shineth
> The everlasting Light;
> The hopes and fears of all the years
> Are met in thee to-night.

My hope was that the next day I would wake up with perfectly normal eyes. But I knew I would not. My hope also was that the next day I would wake up, and my grandmother would be nicer to my mother.

My grandmother rarely hugged Momma or Billy or me, although she did do whatever Billy wanted, because he was the only boy around. I don't think she ever said she loved us. Momma hugged Billy and me all the time, and always said she loved us. I loved Momma most of the time.

"I am going upstairs now," I said. I walked through the hall and smelled the evergreen of the Christmas tree. I pulled off a needle to chew. The other needles pricked my fingers, but the smell of evergreen was wonderful. I climbed up three steps to a landing, thirteen steps to a landing, and five steps to the front hall. I made my way to the little front bedroom I'd slept in as a younger child. A small four-poster doll bed with its canopy missing stood in one corner. Tiny Tears lay in this bed, and I felt her perfectly shaped eyes. Then I felt the child's dresser, with the mirror attached above it. If only I could see in the mirror. Sighted people seemed to look in mirrors all the time to evaluate how they appeared. I decided to go into the middle bedroom. In there, my grandmother kept her unwanted Christmas presents from years gone by. She gave these presents to other people. I wondered what would happen if Grandmomma gave back to a person the exact same gift that person had given her. I smelled bars of scented soap. I felt boxes wrapped in cellophane and shook them and knew they were bottles of cologne. I could hear liquid sloshing inside, and they smelled good. I walked into the front bedroom that Billy and I now shared at Christmas time.

"Not that it matters," Grandmomma had said, "But don't tell anyone that you and Billy share the same room here."

I touched the fireplace. It shared a chimney with the fireplace below, in the living room. Billy entered the room and said he was back from David's, and that he had to put out cookies and juice for Santa. I'd been surprised to find out at school that year that there was no Santa. Most of us had believed in Santa for a long time.

"I wish we had heard from Daddy this Christmas," I said.

"Well, I remember last summer he said he was getting married again and moving to Africa," Billy said. That summer, Daddy had brought me a gold charm that he'd bought at Tiffany's. It was in the shape of a horse.

"I remember Momma had the babysitter stay with us so she wouldn't be at the house when Daddy picked us up. I've always wished Momma and Daddy would get back together."

"I'm going to sleep, Piglet. No point in getting up early."

Silently, I began to tell the story of *"The Night before Christmas"*:

"'Twas the night before Christmas, when all through the house
Not a creature was stirring, not even a mouse;
The stockings were hung by the chimney with care
In hopes that St. Nicholas soon would be there—"

"Hey, Billy, did you hang up the stockings?"

"Yeah. The best things we'll get in them are those gold coins. They're chocolates wrapped up in gold paper."

Oh, yeah, I thought. The coins came in a mesh bag. At least I liked chocolate. But I hated Christmas. Nothing good ever happened at Christmas.

When I woke up and looked outside the next morning, it was still dark. I figured Grandmomma was downstairs drinking prune juice.

"Merry Christmas, Billy," I said. I hoped there were lots of presents downstairs under the Christmas tree, especially presents for me. Billy didn't answer. I felt for and found him in his twin bed and pulled back the covers.

"All right, I'm coming," Billy said. "You're such a pest, Piglet."

Billy jumped out of bed and ran ahead of me down the stairs. I turned left out of the front bedroom and walked down the hall and found the stairway on the right just beyond the cedar chest.

It has always struck me how tedious blindness is in terms of navigating the environment. Sighted people just walk from point A to point B. But blind people memorize and concentrate. I hung on to the banister but walked as quickly as I could down the twenty-one steps to the front hallway.

"Hello, children," Grandmomma said. "Let me go in the kitchen and get you some orange juice."

"Not many presents," Billy whispered.

Grandmomma returned. She put a glass of orange juice wrapped in a paper napkin in my hand. "Don't spill it," she said. I heard Momma's footsteps descend the stairs.

"Mary Jean, go in the powder room and brush your hair."

"Merry Christmas, everyone," Momma said, but she didn't sound happy.

"Here is your small stack of presents," Billy said.

"I've got my yellow legal pad right here so we can write down what we get and write thank-you notes," Grandmomma said.

She reminded me constantly of the importance of thank-you notes. I brought my portable typewriter over there every Christmas and typed my thank-you notes on Christmas afternoon. I showed each letter to Grandmomma, and if I had made one single mistake in the typing, I would have to retype the entire letter at her insistence. It was harder for me than for Billy, because I had a whole page to fill with words I could not proofread. I counted five gifts in my set. I picked up the top one and started unwrapping, one piece of tape at a time.

"Peggy, don't tear that wrapping paper," Grandmomma said. I knew not to tear it. I felt some soap-on-a-rope. It was in a shape of a dog. As usual, the soap smelled like Ivory. "I am sure this is from Miz Buchanan," I said.

"I'm sure it is, but what have you done with the card?" Billy asked. "Oh, here it is," he said. "Merry Christmas from Alice Buchanan."

"Let me see the soap," Grandmomma said. "So I can write it on the pad."

"That soap-on-a-rope is adorable," Momma said.

"Oh, for God Almighty's sake, Alice Buchanan gave me a box of Russell Stover creams. I told her I just like nuts," Grandmomma said.

"Merry Christmas! Merry Christmas!" Clara boomed as I heard her come through the front door. Her brother Bailey drove her to the house on Christmas mornings. His car barely ran. Grandmomma said he was poor as Job's turkey.

"Clara, I have some cards from my friends for you. I am sure they gave you money. I'll bring them to you in the kitchen in a little while."

I thought Clara was lucky. She got to quit school in the fifth grade, and since she couldn't read or write very well, she got to call and thank people instead of writing them thank-you letters.

"You're sitting too close to the tree," Grandmomma said. "Those lights on the bottom string—like the bunch of grapes and the ear of corn—get hotter than the hinges."

I was sitting on the Oriental rug and moved away from the tree. One time I had asked Billy what "hotter than the hinges" meant. He said it meant "hotter than the hinges of Hell."

I smelled a turkey. "Miz Lamson," Clara said. "What time did you put on the turkey?"

"Four a.m.," Grandmomma said.

"I'm gonna change clothes and start breakfast," Clara said.

I was so hoping I would get some nice Christmas presents.

I heard Grandmomma opening a gift. "Victoria gave me a half-slip," she sighed. "It's too small. I'll put it in my bedroom. Well, a pox upon her."

Immediately I thought about the middle bedroom with all the presents to be re-gifted. Later I asked Billy what "a pox upon her" meant.

"I think it means wishing the plague on someone," Billy said. "I think it comes from a play written by that guy Shakespeare."

Then Beany knocked an ornament off a low branch of the Christmas tree. She shook her collar and walked into the living room and lay down on the Oriental rug out there. I picked up another gift from my small stack. I bent the gift back and forth. It felt like socks. Billy read the card and said it was from Santa.

I wanted to cry, but I'd taught myself not to. I had to be strong.

"Christmas makes me tired." Grandmomma said, "December twenty-sixth is my favorite day of the year."

"I got some Gold Cup socks from Santa," Billy said. "Listen, we have to finish opening these presents. David and I want to play football before lunch." My other gifts turned out to be a pair of bedroom slippers, a short silky nightgown, and a red hair bow that I'd never put in my hair. The other kids always made fun of the way I placed bows in my hair.

"Peggy, go tell Clara to come sweep up this broken ornament."

I made my way to the kitchen. The turkey smelled delicious. "Hey, Clara," I said. I heard her banging pots and pans in the sink.

"Hey, darlin'," Clara said and put her arms around me.

I immediately felt better. Clara acted the same all the time.

"Have a seat on the five-cornered wooden stool," Clara said. I heard her pull the heavy stool across the linoleum floor. Clara had told me one time the floor was green.

"What's for Christmas dinner?" I asked.

"We're having turkey and dressing and cranberry sauce, and rice and gravy, and corn cut off the cob, and okra–and-tomato gumbo. The corn looks good. Not as good as Daddy's corn he raised on the farm near Augusta. I used to go pick the corn and string beans and cotton and tobacco. Of course, I came to live with my cousin Ruby when I was fourteen here in Jacksonville. She got me a job with her at Mr. Watson's laundry, and your grandmother met me there. It was always hot in the laundry, and it is always hot in this kitchen. It's that gas stove."

"Did you like working at the laundry, Clara?"

"Sure, I did. Mr. Watson taught me how to sleeve shirts and put a ring around the collar. Your grandmother said she liked my work, and if I would come work for her she would be happy. I have been working for her for forty years."

I loved stories. I sometimes tried to remember when I first realized I was blind. I think it was when I was about four, when I ran the doll carriage into the new chair in Houston and poked a hole in the upholstery.

"I used to drive my daddy's wagon to church," Clara said. "Mount Carmel Baptist Church in Appling, Georgia. I sat up high and drove that horse and wagon. I'm a country woman. The rest of the family sat in the back in chairs and straw. As we drove along, we sang, 'Jesus, Keep Me Near the Cross.'"

"Sing it for me, Clara."

"Jesus, keep me near the cross," Clara began to sing. "Very precious master..." Then, "I don't remember it all."

***

The summer after my third-grade year, it was 1963, my mother began a master's degree in English at the University of Florida. She said she was tired of teaching junior-high music. So, while Billy went to summer camp at Camp Greenville in South Carolina, Momma and I went to Gainesville so she could begin her studies.

When we first got to our apartment, Momma told me it consisted of a living room, a bedroom, a bathroom and a kitchen. Then she said she was going to the grocery store and left.

I had spent some time walking into walls and cabinets, trying to figure out the layout of the apartment, when the phone rang. I found it, picked it up, and said, "Hello?"

"Hello, Peggy," my grandmother said. "Where is your mother?"

"She went to the grocery store," I said.

"Oh, for God's sake. Does she have any sense of responsibility, leaving you there alone? I am coming down there right now."

My mother wouldn't like that. When she got back, I told her Grandmomma was on her way, and would be there in about an hour.

"Oh, no," Momma said. "I can't stand it. I hate my mother. And I saw a man at the store who looked somewhat like your father. Reminded me of stories. I just have to scream, or I have to laugh."

Then she said, "Let me tell you something." She was speaking very loudly. "Your father and I were living in Wyoming, and he was a roustabout in an oil field. One day he stepped on a rusty nail. There was no place for me to take him except the hospital. They gave him a tetanus shot but wanted to keep him overnight. So, I took my Dalmatian, Brucey, to a hotel with me and checked in. I did not lock the door to my hotel room. I just got in bed because I was tired and pregnant with Billy. I started reading an article by J. Edgar Hoover. He said that if a drunk man wandered into your hotel room in the middle of the night, you should be perfectly still. And then a drunk man walked into my hotel room, and I was perfectly still. Brucey didn't even wake up. And then the man wandered out and back into the hall. I didn't tell your father about it. Your father would have been so angry."

But Momma just started laughing and laughing.

I know now that she was in a manic phase of bipolar disorder, signified by all the laughter. The poor judgment she described in the story may have been part of the disease as well. But at the time, this was just another example of her puzzling behavior. One of Momma's outbursts. It was far from the last.

One day, a distant cousin named Mary and I took the bus into town to go shopping. While we were out, Mary said, "I'll make you a muumuu. Let's get some material and a pattern."

I didn't have any cash except for my return bus fare. Mary bought the material and the pattern and said it came to $1.21 total. This was in 1963.

When I got home, I told Momma in front of Mary about the $1.21. Momma blew up. She said I never should have borrowed the money and that all she had planned to give me was bus fare. Anyway, she paid Mary, and I hid the material and the pattern in the bottom of a drawer.

Stress of any kind, including financial stress, can trigger bipolar episodes. Momma, who'd been brought up in a relatively wealthy family, was now a divorced schoolteacher with two kids. She was relying on the generosity of her aunt to pay for her master's degree. Meanwhile, her brilliant but alcoholic ex-husband kept losing his jobs and didn't pay child support.

As Billy and I would one day understand, Momma's anger was part of her disorder. Moreover, bipolar disorder never goes away. Not long ago, I was visiting Momma in her new apartment in the retirement community, and she said for me to have a seat at the kitchen table. I asked her which seat I should sit in. She said I could sit anywhere I goddamn well pleased.

I felt hurt and shocked but sat down. There really wasn't anywhere for me to go.

Chapter Seven

We were living in Jacksonville the summer after I turned eleven. It was 1963. Momma surprised me with an early birthday present—a bicycle built for two. It was a gleaming, red-and-white Schwinn. Momma suggested that Billy or my good friend Jacky ride on the front and that I ride on the back. Billy took me for a spin, and I quickly realized the person on the back didn't have to pedal. But the person in front got to steer.

The next day Jacky was coming over. I had walked the bike to the end of our driveway and parked it in the shade of our old oak tree. I could see that the front seat was red, and I was planning to ride on it. I heard the tires of a bike, probably Jacky's, bumping up and down on the sidewalk and coming toward me. There were bumps in the sidewalk because the roots of the old oak tree had pushed it up. Jacky called, "Hi."

"Look at my bike!" I shouted.

"Beautiful!" Jacky exclaimed.

She sounded very close to me now. "I have never seen a bicycle built for two except on TV."

"Can I ride on the front and you ride on the back, Jacky, and give directions?"

"Sure," Jacky said. "Where do you want to go?"

"Let's go to Park and King and get a chocolate double-dip ice cream cone," I said.

I mounted the bike and listened for Jacky to situate herself on the back. My shorts and shirt were already starting to stick to me in the Florida heat. "You ready, Jacky?"

"Yes!"

"Let's go!" I shouted, and I steered toward the driveway and to the left. The bike wobbled.

"You're doing okay," Jacky said. "Steer on down into the street. Too many tree roots in the sidewalk."

I turned right on my street, Herschel, which headed toward the park. "I hate the smell of mosquito spray," I said. The truck had come the night before. "You are going past the corner," Jacky said. "Turn right."

I made the turn and almost dumped the bike over, but I was determined to keep going. We were riding down Willow Branch Avenue with houses on our right and a park on our left. Occasionally we rode through the shade of an oak tree. "Here is Riverside Avenue," Jacky said. "Turn left."

So, I turned onto Riverside Avenue. Cars whizzed by at top speed. I struggled to keep the bike upright. "Steer to your left," Jacky shouted. "Here comes a truck!"

I steered to the left. The truck roared safely by. I was focused.

"Here is Oak Street," Jacky said. "Turn left."

I did. Oak Street had much less traffic than Riverside Avenue. "Do you have fifteen cents for an ice cream cone?" Jacky asked me.

"Yeah, I have a quarter."

Just then I felt my left handle bar grip slide down the side of a car, which was bad but at least my hand wasn't caught.

"You kids!" A man yelled. "That is my brand-new black Mustang! Look at the white streak your handlebar grip made! I am calling your parents. What are your phone numbers?"

"But I'm blind!" I cried. "I didn't see your car!"

"You get on the back of that bike. Your friend who can see should get on the front. You all just run along."

I felt my way to the back of the bike. I tried to look helpless and hung my head. At least I wouldn't have to pedal. Jacky got on the front. Soon we had turned a corner. I said, "That man can't see us now. Let me back on the front of the bike."

We switched places. We were off again. "We're passing Azalea Terrace on the right," Jacky said. "Just cross on over."

"I need you to pedal, Jacky," I said.

"Just one more block 'til Park and King. I can't wait for my chocolate ice cream cone," she said.

Many years later I asked Momma if she knew I used to ride on the front of the tandem bike. She said she didn't, but I feel sure somebody must have given her a call. That first bike ride was far from our last, and I often insisted on steering. Someone once told me my biggest interpersonal issue is a need to be in control; I'm sure that's true. Somehow, I ended up taking after my grandmother in that way. Also, as a blind child I learned to be aggressive—to attack the environment rather than hide from it. Jacky was fairly patient with my bossiness, but on at least one occasion we got into an argument about it.

We were in the wooden porch swing on Grandmomma's side porch. "Where do you wanna eat lunch today?" Jacky asked.

"Let's go to your apartment and have a tuna fish sandwich," I said.

"I want to stay here and have Clara's cooking," Jacky said. "What's she fixing for lunch today?"

"Pork chop casserole with sweet potatoes, apples, onions, and rice and gravy."

"That sounds great," Jacky said. "Who wants a tuna fish sandwich?"

"But we always eat here. I want to eat at your place sometimes. Besides, your mother is at work. If we eat here, we'll have to eat with my grandmother. She'll tell me to chew with my mouth closed, and use my biscuit to push with instead of my fingers. And she'll ask why I don't grow my hair nice and long like yours." I reached out and felt thin air. Then I moved my hand closer to where I knew Jacky sat and felt her long, curly hair.

"All right," Jacky said, "Have it your way. And I'm sure you want to ride on the front."

"Of course," I said.

It was the week after Christmas. It had been three years since Granddaddy died. John F. Kennedy had been assassinated just before

Thanksgiving. We walked the bike across Riverside Avenue because of all the traffic. Then we hopped on and rode the five blocks to Jacky's apartment. I heard Jacky's key turn in the lock, and we walked into the living room. It occurred to me that my mother never locked our doors. The apartment smelled new. "Momma painted our living room white, and she bought a black couch," Jacky said.

As I sank into the deep carpet, I grabbed Jacky's arm. I was sure there was a coffee table to walk around. I held on to Jacky's arm until we reached the hard floor of the kitchen. Jacky put my hand on the back of a kitchen chair, which I knew had a padded seat. I held my head up and turned my face toward the outside light. I knew I was looking at a wall of windows. I heard Jacky opening a can and smelled the delicious aroma of tuna fish.

"Put some pickle relish in it," I cried.

"I don't like pickle relish," she said. "You're so bossy, Peggy."

"Well, just put the pickle relish in mine," I said. "You like mayonnaise, don't you?"

"We always have to do what you want to do because you're blind," Jacky said.

"Do not!"

"Do so!" Jacky said.

"I do not get my way all the time," I said. "I wanted four new dresses for Christmas, and I didn't get any. Listen, Jacky, you're being rude. My grandmother says never to be rude to guests. Anyway, I don't want any tuna fish or pickle relish. I'm taking my bike and walking home."

I was going to point out that I thought Jacky's mother wore too much perfume, but I decided not to do that.

I made it through the living room, around the coffee table and out the front door. I let myself out. No steps. With my foot I found the grass-sidewalk line. I followed the sidewalk until I felt my bike. I pulled up the kickstand. On the main sidewalk I started walking the bike toward home. It was heavy and unwieldy because it was a tandem. Occasionally, I came upon breaks in the sidewalk where tree roots had broken through.

Walking under trees or out in the open felt about the same because it was winter, and there was no shade. It was a cool day, and I felt fine in my long-sleeved shirt. I carefully stopped at corners and listened for cars. I crossed five streets and made it to my street, Herschel, where Billy, Momma, and I lived. That night Jacky called to see if I had made it. "Sure did," I said.

Jacky could see, but she never saw her father. At least Daddy came to see Billy and me once in a while.

I started thinking about the fact that my tandem bike had a lot of red on it. Since red was the only color I could see, I was glad my bike was partly red. I knew I was blinded by red devil lye, but I didn't know what red devil lye came in: would it be a bottle or a jar? Kids said my left eye looked kind of red and so the false eye maker painted my false eye to look kind of red. Doctor K. always gave me a red lollipop after my eye exam and Grandmomma was taking me to see him next week.

***

I sat in the chair in Dr. K.'s small exam room and inhaled the scent of clean air. Grandmomma sat across from me. She always had to be involved in any doctor's appointment. Dr. K. came in with a hearty "hello" and just looked at my eye with a flashlight.

"Can you make my eyes look better?" I asked. "I just want to be pretty."

"'Pretty is as pretty does'" he said.

I never liked that saying. I guess it meant you were pretty if you did good things but I did good things like pet the dog, and pet the cat, and set the table for supper, and wash dishes, and kids still made fun of my eyes, so it didn't make me pretty.

***

One time when I was in high school, I had on a fitted dress when I went to an appointment with Dr. K. He said I looked great, which surprised me but also pleased me. My eye with the prosthesis was swollen, making the prosthesis protrude unnaturally. Several of my friends at school had commented on it, and asked if anything could be done. I was worried and scared. Momma acted oblivious to the whole thing. I asked Dr. K why my eye was protruding so much.

He said, "Your eye has a hernia, which is causing the prosthesis to protrude."

That's all he said, so I guess he was just looking at me in the dress. He no longer offered me a red lollipop, but his office still smelled fresh and clean.

Also in high school, my grandmother took me to Dr. K.'s for an appointment. She had to go somewhere, and he said he would take me home. I wore what I had been told were yellow shorts and a yellow shirt. I had long, very straight blonde hair. Dr. K surprised me after a quick look at my left eye with a flashlight. He didn't even ask if I could still see light, dark, or the color red. Instead, he invited me back into his private office. I heard him lock the door after we went in. He led me over to a very large, soft, and comfortable sofa. Then he said he thought I had a great body.

"But you are married!" I exclaimed.

"That's all right," he said. "I see other women, particularly at medical conventions out of town."

I was stunned.

"But what about your wife?" I cried.

"What about her?" he responded. And he reached over and caressed one of my nipples.

"I think I want to go home," I said.

"Okay," he said. "I have a new Cadillac Seville. But give some thought to coming back soon."

I just wanted out of there. One of the drawbacks of being blind is you have to hold on to other people to get out of an unfamiliar room. I couldn't just bolt.

I didn't tell anyone about this situation until some years later.

***

At age 11, Momma asked me to take piano lessons. She said Mrs. Hoskins would come to our house every Wednesday from 4:00 to 4:30 to teach me. Momma played the piano so well, and I didn't know how good I would be.

I remembered Mr. Hoskins had been her harmony teacher when she was 19, and she failed his class. Then last year, while she finished her music degree at age 35 at Jacksonville University, she had Mr. Hoskins for her harmony teacher again, and she made an A. He told her she was a very musical person.

Anyway, I suffered through about 15 piano lessons and hated to practice. Momma made me practice 15 minutes a day from 5:30 to 5:45 every afternoon. For such a laid-back parent, Momma could be amazingly stern and strict at times.

Finally, I spoke sharply to Mrs. Hoskins during a lesson. I said, "I just don't like playing the piano. In fact, I hate playing the piano. I just do it for Momma. I wish I could be one of those great blind musicians, but I can't."

At that point, I heard Momma's footsteps walking across the dining room and into the living room where Mrs. Hoskins and I sat on the bench of the baby grand piano. "Peggy, watch your tone of voice," she said.

"I've been thinking she doesn't much like playing the piano," Mrs. Hoskins said.

"Would it be best if she quit taking piano lessons?" Momma asked.

"Yes, Momma," I interrupted. "I like creative writing."

***

One night at age eleven I pretended to be asleep when I heard Momma walk quietly into my room. She slid the phone across the dresser. She closed the door as best she could but could not close it completely because of the phone cord. I heard her walk into the kitchen and set the phone base on the kitchen table. On a rotary dial phone, I could hear the short sounds of twos and threes being dialed and the long sounds of sevens, eights, and nines being dialed.

"Shirley?" Momma asked quietly.

Pause.

"I'm just so jealous of so many teachers. 'Specially the teachers who have husbands. And they talk about their husbands all the time. And all those teachers have newer cars than I have. I have the oldest car in the parking lot."

"The other day," Momma went on, "my mother said she couldn't believe I had been a debutante and didn't marry a doctor or lawyer and live in Ortega as all the others in my debutante coterie have done."

Pause.

"Well, thank you, Shirley. You're a good friend."

"I just hate so many people and I'm so jealous of so many people. Anne is this beautiful young teacher who everybody likes. I just hate her."

Pause.

"Someone said I was beautiful? Well, then they need their eyes examined."

I cringed in bed. The beauty thing again. "Listen, Shirley, I think I'm going crazy. I know this is strange, but I can't help it. I'll drive toward a green light and think that if I can get through it while it is still green, I will live. If it turns red before I can get through it, I will die."

Pause.

"Yes, I do talk to my psychiatrist. He just tells me to take my medication and come in every two weeks. I hope my children know I love them."

As an adult, I have rarely heard my mother talk this openly about her unhappiness. Recently she has talked about suicide. She has said she would jump in front of a car or jump in the river, but I have talked to her psychiatrist, and he does not think she would do so. She has occasionally checked into psych wards, but usually within a day or two she has been released. It is so hard that at times Momma is negative about everything. Her psychiatrist says she has got to get her mind off herself.

***

Sometimes Paul's mother took us to the beach. Paul was the only other blind kid I knew. He was one year ahead of me in elementary school, finishing up sixth grade as I was finishing up fifth. Every other kid in our elementary school of 600 students was sighted.

I remember one particular Saturday when Paul's mother and Paul and his little sister, Paulette, picked me up at my house. I didn't take any suntan lotion although I loved the smell of it. We were headed to the beach. I knew I was going to get sunburned. When we got to the beach, Mrs. Kurtz found a spot near the water where Paul and I could sit on the sand and build a sandcastle. I drizzled some sand on a spot between us, and Paul did as well. Our hands met.

"They're holding hands, Momma," Paul's little sister screamed.

Then I drizzled sand and avoided Paul's hand. The seagulls shrieked, and the surf roared. The sun felt like heaven on my face. My bottom was creating a seat for me in the wet sand.

"Let's go in the water," Paul said.

I knew he stood up because his voice came from above me. "Come on, come on," he said as I followed him into the water.

"Don't go too far," Paul's mother yelled.

I followed Paul's voice, which continued to lead me out into the water. "Let's stop here," he said when we were waist-deep between waves.

We put our hands under water and held hands again. I was glad he had a hard hand and not a soft one.

"Let's duck under the next wave, and I'll kiss you," he said.

We ducked under the next wave and while it passed over, Paul followed up my arm with his hand and over my shoulder to my face. He held onto me with one hand and found my mouth with his other hand and kissed me. After he did, I swallowed some salt water. I hope nobody saw that.

"I don't think sighted people can see into ocean water. They sure can see a lot though. How did you like the kiss?" Paul asked.

"I liked it," I said. "Let's do it again."

And so, we did. After a little while we followed the waves to shore. I held on to Paul's arm so we could stay together. Paul's mother met us in the shallow water and said, "Come and have lunch." She suggested I hold on to one of her arms and that Paul hold on to the other. She guided us back to dry ground and a big beach towel on the sand. We sat together while we ate fried chicken and baked beans and drank lemonade. The sun shone down, and the breeze blew. The fried chicken tasted good but not as good as Clara's.

"Do you want to go to the Schoolboy Safety Patrol dance with me?" Paul asked.

"Yes, thank you."

I wondered what Grandmomma would think of that. She referred to Paul as "the blind boy." She said we looked a lot alike. But then I remembered neither of us knew how to dance. Maybe we could sit on the sidelines and listen to music and drink Cokes.

When I got home, I told Momma I'd had a great time with Paul and wanted to go the Schoolboy Patrol Dance with him.

"Wonderful, peach cake," she said.

I figured life would be very hard if I married a blind person.

***

When I was in the fifth grade at Central Riverside, I was asked to be the mistress of ceremonies at the dedication of a garden for the blind. I guess because two blind kids, Paul and I, attended this school, the Jacksonville Garden Club decided we should have a garden for the blind on the front grounds of our school. They grew plants with interesting shaped leaves and aromas in the garden and placed metal Braille name tags on each plant. They put pathways in the garden so we could identify them as we walked through. They included a concrete pathway, a pathway of pebbles, a pathway of pine straw, and one with three big stepping stones leading to a bird feeder. In general, I didn't like attention being called to my blindness, but I was mesmerized by the garden and the paths.

On dedication day, when I got to speak to the crowd, I wore a peach-colored dress with lace I could feel at the neck and on the ends of the short sleeves. I spoke about the different pathways and the different aromas of the plants. I broke in half a citrus leaf and inhaled its lovely aroma and described it to the crowd. I broke in half a eucalyptus leaf and reacted negatively to its terrible smell.

Great applause followed my speech. Grandmomma, who was a high achiever, praised me to the skies, especially when the story was written up in the newspaper. Momma just gave me a big hug and said, "I love you, peach cake."

In retrospect, I still like the garden for the blind and the ceremony where I spoke. The chance to be a star overrode any concerns about blindness.

***

One day when I was in the sixth grade my mother said my grandmother was not at home. Clara was at her house and Momma wanted me to walk over there. She wanted me to carry a large silver water pitcher she wanted Clara to polish. I had on what I knew was a short navy and white summer dress and sandals. Momma put the big silver pitcher in my hand, and I made my way out the front door and counted down the five front porch steps. I never counted steps when I walked on flat ground. But because of practice, I knew how to walk across the front walkway from the bottom of the five steps to the small step that led to the main sidewalk. I turned left and by practice knew where big roots were pushing up the sidewalk. I easily avoided the spot.

It was a hot humid summer day, but we had so many trees on our block that the shade cut the heat somewhat. The old sidewalk felt rough even when tree roots didn't break it up. I knew I was passing Mrs. Christy's house—she lived next to us—until the rough sidewalk gave way to the smoothness of her concrete driveway. The silver pitcher weighed a lot, but I continued. I crossed over Mrs. Corde's driveway, and on the other side I put my hand on Mrs. Bisbee's fence. People had told me it was white. Following the picket fence to the corner, I turned left and made my way to the alley and crossed. After passing the Hazlehurst house and crossing a quiet Oak Street, I reassured myself of my location by touching a U.S. mailbox on my right.

As an adult, I realize how much more laborious the world of a blind person is compared to that of a sighted person. A sighted person can just stand at one end of the block and look at the other end and walk straight there.

A blind person has to concentrate heavily when moving around. I paused at the mailbox and put the silver pitcher in my other hand. Walking again, I could hear the traffic ahead of me on Riverside Avenue. I would have to cross Riverside Avenue and then a quiet street, McDuff, in order to reach my grandmother's. Just when I was preparing to cross Riverside, the elastic in my underwear popped. My underwear fell to my feet, and I was mortified. I stepped out of my underwear and threw it into the silver pitcher.

My grandmother did not like my crossing Riverside Avenue by myself, but she wasn't at home. I listened for a lull in traffic and crossed Riverside, then quickly crossed McDuff. I put my hand on a low stone wall that ran in front of the Loves' house. It was pointed, and I liked to walk on it with my feet on either side of the point. However, right now, I had the silver pitcher. I knew next I would walk by Mrs. Taylor's house with the scent of many flowering shrubs. Then the Studts' with their barking dog. Finally, I reached my grandmother's driveway, which had a sidewalk running in front of it but was paved with leaves. I had made it safely here and was taking the silver pitcher inside to Clara.

***

The next day I was at my grandmother's again and my grandmother and I were in her sitting room. I sprawled on the sofa, which I knew by touch had on its summer slipcover. The phone rang. Clara picked it up in the breakfast room on the other side of the swinging door. "Hello!" she shouted.

"For forty years I have asked Clara to answer the phone 'Lamson residence' and for forty years she has said, 'Hello.' It irritates my soul."

I heard Clara say, "Thank you. Good bye." Then I heard the swinging door open. "Miz Lamson, that was Miz Morris. She said the bridge game would be at her house. It will be tomorrow at 1:30 instead of 1:00. She said she won't be back from the beauty parlor before 1:15."

"Thank you, Clara. Next time answer the phone 'Lamson residence.'"

Clara didn't say anything.

As an adult, I'm struck by how different life was for grandmother and her crowd than it is for most of the women I know today. Grandmomma's friends all had servants. They didn't work. They went to the beauty parlor all the time or went to the Garden Club or played bridge. Actually, for even my mother to work in her generation was out of the norm. But she was divorced, so she had to work.

"Your mother needs her hair done, Peggy," my grandmother said. "She doesn't notice it. She doesn't notice your false eye. I don't understand your mother. I don't understand anything."

"Grandmomma, can you tell me a story? Maybe about when you were in college?"

"I went to college in Louisburg, West Virginia. I was eighteen. The college was called Greenbrier Seminary for Girls. That was in 1915. I took the train up there from Jacksonville. It was an all-girls college, and we could only have dates on Monday afternoon in the parlor from two to four o'clock. I had a beau named Felix who gave me a lavaliere. This happened on a Monday afternoon—I'm saving it for you. In 1916, after my freshman year of college, my sister Mary died. She went out on a day cruise and came down with appendicitis. She was only sixteen. After Mary died, Mother wanted me to come home, and I did. Mother wore black every day for the rest of her life."

Clara had told me that my great grandmother was the meanest white woman she ever knew. The only good thing she ever did for Clara was teach her how to cook shrimp pilau.

"I am going to get that lavaliere right now and give it to you," Grandmomma said. I heard her walk over to the secretary and pull out a drawer. Then she closed the drawer. As she walked over to me, I held out my hand. I held my hand at exactly the right moment and didn't have to leave it hanging out there.

The lavaliere was a small, intricate piece of jewelry with a stone in the middle. "I think the stone is a peridot," Grandmomma said. "I want you to have it, Peggy."

It struck me that, perhaps in her own way, my grandmother did love me.

***

In the fifth grade I took ballet. Everyone else in the class was in the third grade and could see. Mrs. Baggs came and positioned my feet in first, second, third, fourth, and fifth so I could learn the positions. We often worked at the barre. But I hated standing out. I just wanted to blend in. We all wore black leotards and pink tights. My grandmother took me and picked me up.

For the end of the year recital, we were doing the ballet of Dick Whittington. I was a rat. For my costume I wore a brown satin leotard with fur at the top. I had a long brown tail and brown taffeta ears.

The day after the recital we got some very sad news. The body of my little cousin Walter washed up on the banks of the St. Johns River. He was six years old and had been missing for three days.

When Walter was two, Momma, Billy, and I babysat him at the beach for six weeks while his parents and older siblings went on a trip around the world. We stayed in the family's beach house, so I felt close to him. When Walter first went missing, the family thought he had been kidnapped. Some prominent men of Jacksonville spent a night at a bank counting out a million dollars in small bills that could be used as ransom money. It was 1964.

Alas, Walter had walked out on the dock in his family's backyard. He fell in the river and drowned. It was my first experience with death other than my grandfather's. Again, I found death very sad.

I loved to go to Evergreen Cemetery; it reminded me that one day I would die and be buried there. Momma always said not to stand on the graves. Sometimes I knelt beside a grave and felt the carving in the tombstone. My great-great grandfather J. J. Daniel had a monument with a bench around it. He had been a prominent Jacksonville lawyer (not a doctor) and a Colonel in the Civil War. He died in the yellow fever epidemic in Jacksonville in 1888.

***

One day in sixth grade I made my usual summer evening walk

over to the Wheelers'. Beany trotted along behind me. The Wheelers lived next door to us. I always walked straight to Mr. Wheeler because I could hear the sound of his hose which he used to water his lawn. I used to walk through his grass in the daytime when it was dry and thick and lush until he asked me not to walk through it anymore.

Beany jingled the tags on her collar. "Hello, Peggy, hello, Beany," Mr. Wheeler said over the sound of the spraying water.

"I'm going to turn the hose off now. I'll get you a red lollipop and Beany some vanilla wafers."

Beany and I made our way to his red brick front porch and climbed the three steps. I knew there were two wrought-iron chairs on either side of the porch, and I sat down in one. Beany flopped on the front porch beside me. In those days dogs ate anything. In a few minutes the screen door opened, and Mr. Wheeler said, "Beany, here you go!"

I heard Beany chomp on her vanilla wafers, and I heard her toenails click as she ran off the porch. Mr. Wheeler put a lollipop in my hand. It was the kind with the curled stem; he had taken off the wrapper.

"Mrs. Wheeler has gone to play bridge," he said. "By the way, a girl needs three things. She needs a good personality, a good brain, and a good figure. You have the personality and the brain. I always enjoy talking to you. You are a straight A student. But you need to gain some weight. Do you know how much you weigh?"

"Not really," I said. "But I sure do eat a lot of Clara's fried chicken and rice and gravy."

I liked Mr. Wheeler. I didn't talk to him about being blind. That word just seemed so scary and complicated to me. But I talked to him about how I did in school. "Come inside," Mr. Wheeler said, "and I will weigh you. Then you can weigh here once a week."

I didn't think anything of it. I had gotten lollipops from Mr. Wheeler for the last five years, and Beany had gotten vanilla wafers. I carried my lollipop, and Mr. Wheeler guided me through the house to the downstairs bathroom. "Step on the scale," he said. "99 pounds."

I had on peach-colored shorts and a peach-and-white print blouse. Momma had told me. I also wore flip-flops. It smelled like some kind of food had been cooked in his house, but I couldn't identify it.

"You can step off the scale," Mr. Wheeler said and put his hand on my breast. I had not yet started wearing a bra. He left it there for a few seconds then took it away and said, "I'm not supposed to do this."

I didn't say anything. And I didn't tell my mother. I wasn't sure what she would say or do. I was sort of scared.

Beany and I went over for a lollipop and vanilla wafers far less often, and I never went in Mr. Wheeler's house again.

As an adult, I wonder why I didn't tell my mother. She would not have overreacted. I don't think I ever told anybody about the incident.

***

On a Saturday morning just two weeks later, my friend Carol and I were walking home from spending the night with my Uncle Dick. He lived in a huge house on the river and was at least 90 years old. He had a fulltime nurse. There were some intriguing things about Uncle Dick's situation. His butler, Wilbur, and his cook Viola, made the best silver dollar pancakes. They fought like cats and dogs in the kitchen while they were making them. Wilbur also served as Uncle Dick's chauffeur. He drove him around Jacksonville in a Volkswagen Beetle. This did not seem like appropriate transportation to me for a retired lawyer. Anyway, we walked home singing "When you're happy and you know it, clap your hands."

***

The seventh grade stood out for me. I attended the same junior high where Billy was in the ninth grade and Momma taught English.

My homeroom teacher and my math teacher were the same person, Mrs. Weyland. The first day during home room Mrs. Weyland had a student walk me to the classroom next door. We walked into the room, and I heard the rustle of paper. I thought the student who brought me was handing the teacher, Miss Taylor, a note.

"Oh," Miss Taylor said, and took me by the hand and led me to a desk. I put out my hand and felt where to sit.

"You will be staying here a little while," Miss Taylor said.

I thought Mrs. Weyland was talking to my class about me and my blindness. My heart sank. Miss Taylor began talking to her homeroom class about school rules. Eventually, a student came back for me. I held on to her arm, but she didn't walk wide enough for two when we went out of the classroom door, and I bumped my shoulder on the doorframe. It really hurt, but I said it didn't.

We went into Mrs. Weyland's class, it was absolutely silent. That is the worst thing that can happen to a blind person when entering a room. I needed somebody to say something. I tripped on the leg of a desk trying to get into it, and I felt my cheeks grow red and hot. I felt so embarrassed and worried about the whole morning.

I had math that day with Mrs. Weyland in the last period of the day. After class she detained me and said she wanted to talk to me about my upcoming math tests. She said she would have me come up and sit at her desk; she would quietly call out the questions, and I could quietly give my answers. I decided I would make a hundred on every math test, and I did.

***

One Sunday both Billy and Momma were sick, so I was the only one who went to Sunday school. My grandmother said she would take me, and while I was at Sunday school, she would have a Bloody Mary with her sister-in-law, Varina. Then she would pick me up afterward. Soon, I heard her horn honk and her Rambler idling at the curb. I crossed the front porch, counted five steps down, continued down the walkway, stepped onto the sidewalk and crossed over it, then crossed the sparse grass to Grandmomma's car. I found the front doorhandle on the passenger's side, opened it carefully, stepped off the curb into the car, and sat down. We had no seatbelts in those days.

"Is Lover Poo tossed in the backseat?" I asked.

"Yes," Grandmomma said, but she didn't sound happy.

I knew that was a bad sign. I was trying to figure out if Grandmomma was mad at me about something or if she was mad at my mother for something like being seen at a department store in blue jeans with holes in them. Grandmomma pulled quickly into the street and headed for Willow Branch Avenue. She said, "Why did you wear that short-waist dress with maroon flowers? And that straw hat with the black ribbon looks dreadful. I bought you that nice yellow linen dress with the multicolored jacket to wear to church. Why didn't you wear that?"

"I wore it last week. But take me home, Grandmomma, and I'll change clothes."

Grandmomma had already driven down Willow Branch Avenue and turned onto Riverside Avenue. I knew the layout because I walked and biked these streets all the time.

"I don't have time," Grandmomma said. "I don't dare be late to

Varina's for a Bloody Mary."

"Momma said I looked cute," I said defensively.

"I have told you and told you that your mother doesn't notice anything. She just reads books and listens to music. She has no taste in clothes."

As an adult, I would use a certain term for my grandmother's behavior here. The term is "double binding." She told me I looked bad and should be wearing something else. Yet she wouldn't take me back home to change.

"That straw hat you have on really makes the outfit," Grandmomma said sarcastically, "but just leave it on."

And then there was my false eye. I knew it didn't look completely natural, and I felt bad about it.

"Am I almost at church?" I asked.

"Yes, you are."

"Thank you," I said.

"I'll pick you up in front of the Sunday school building at eleven-fifteen."

Well, I knew one thing. I'd know every answer that the Sunday school teacher asked the class. The previous week, teacher named Mr. Gardiner, had asked me to quit raising my hand, answering all the questions, and let somebody else have a chance to answer something.

***

Still in 7th grade—I won the school-wide spelling bee at Lake Shore Junior High School. This meant I could go to the county bee.

I called and told my elderly cousins, Theodora and Mary, the good news. They offered to pick me up several times a week after school and take me to their apartment. They wanted to call out all the words in the practice spelling book so I could learn to spell them.

What was interesting about Theodora and Mary were their eccentricities. The afternoon after I called them, Mary and Theodora picked me up. They rang our front doorbell. It was at least 100 degrees in Florida in May, and they asked if I needed my coat. Mary said she had on her pink summer coat with a turquoise straw hat. She said she spray-painted a kitchen chair turquoise and used the rest of the paint to spray the hat. Theodora said she had on a white summer coat and a straw hat.

I carried my practice spelling book with me and Mary helped me into what I knew was a white station wagon. Momma called it the "white peril" because Mary constantly put on the brakes. When Mary put on the brakes, I could hear water sloshing in huge bottles in the bed of the station wagon. These were left over from the Cuban missile crisis which occurred three years previously. While Mary braked and the water sloshed, Theodora recited poetry.

> "'Oh, to be a turtle,
> A slow lethargic turtle
> With nothing in this world to do
> But crawl around the whole day through
> Among the reeds and rushes cool
> To sit for hours on a log
> And gossip idly with a frog
> And think no matter what befell
> I could just crawl into my shell
> And let the whole world go to Pieces.'"

Theodora laughed. I tried to laugh like this was the first time I had heard this poem when in fact it was the fiftieth.

Next on the car ride Theodora began to recite "What would be the result—"

Mary interrupted. "Cousin Theodora, I don't like that."

But Theodora plowed forward.

> "'What would be the result
> If an incoherent heterogeneous homogeneity
> Be resolved in a coherent heterogeneous homogeneity?
> The result would be a barren prolixity of casuistry'".

Brake, slosh, brake slosh.

Mary somehow parked the car. We crossed the sidewalk under the shade of the huge old oak trees. We mounted three steps and entered the foyer of an apartment building. Then we climbed five steps and turned right. In front of us was what I knew was the door to their apartment. I asked if I could ring the bell, which turned like a key in the middle of the door. Of course, no one was there. I rang, and then Mary opened the door with her key. Once inside, I heard them take off their coats and hats. Then they seated me in an armchair with lace antimacassars on the arms. My two cousins never focused on my blindness. They just ignored it.

Mary brought in apricot juice and cookies, and the spelling words began. I had to prepare for the county-wide bee where 50 people would participate.

I successfully spelled antimacassar, unctuous, moratorium, uxoricide, and pantheon. The race was on!

As it turned out, I spelled several words successfully at the county bee. When there were only seventeen participants left out of 50, I misspelled the word "subservient" and was out. The other sixteen made it to the next round.

I was upset, but Momma wasn't. She said just to listen to a book on a talking-book record, and it would get my mind off the spelling bee. She said she always read books when she was upset or depressed.

***

During the summer after I finished 8th grade and Billy finished 10th grade, we flew from Jacksonville to Massachusetts to spend two weeks with our dad. I felt nervous about seeing him. Billy and I had not seen him in over three years, when he stopped by Jacksonville briefly to introduce us to his second wife and their new baby daughter. They were on their way to Africa, where he had been hired by Mobil Oil as a geologist. By then, however, he had lost the job in Africa and divorced his second wife. He was living with his foster mother in her summer mansion in Worthington, Massachusetts, where Billy and I would stay as well.

"What are you doing?" I asked Billy as we sat on the plane.

"I'm reading *To Kill a Mockingbird*. I want to be more like Atticus Finch."

I hadn't read *To Kill a Mockingbird* but thought I would order it on a talking-book record. I wished I could see and could just grab a print book and bring it on an airplane. Very few books come in Braille. As time went on and more and more books were put in audio format, Braille diminished even more.

"Hey Billy," I said, "Do you think I'm above average in intelligence?" I felt the plane dip slightly.

"You're above average in many ways, Piglet. But because you're blind...."

I didn't want to go down that road, so I started thinking about our dad. He was the youngest of five children and the only one born in the United States. His father was from Dresden, and his mother was from London. For some years they lived in Germany, where my grandfather worked for Shroeders Bank. My grandfather came to America in 1921 to set up a U.S. branch of the bank. He arrived as Paul Stephen Schluckwerder. Fortunately for the rest of us, he changed his name to Paul Stephen Paul. When the stock market crashed in 1929, Grandfather Paul became so depressed after losing so much money that he left his wife and children, never to be heard from again. The family lost their house in New York. My grandmother Paul took her family to live in their summer home in Worthington, Massachusetts, in the Berkshires. At this point, Daddy was four.

By the time Daddy was in second grade, his teachers had determined he was highly intelligent. A childless and wealthy couple in Worthington, Roy and Helen McCann, offered to take him in and educate him at their winter home in Scarsdale, New York. By this point, Daddy felt abandoned by both his father and his mother. Ultimately, the McCanns sent Daddy to the Colorado School of Mines and then on to Harvard, where he met our mother, who was attending the Boston Conservatory.

When we landed at Hartford Springfield Airport, I noticed how much cooler it was than when we had left Jacksonville in the summer heat. We got into the back seat of Uncle Allerton's large, comfortable car. It smelled new. He said it was his brand-new Cadillac. Uncle Allerton was a smooth-talking customs lawyer, and he was married to one of Daddy's sisters, my aunt Marjorie. She often spoke sharply and in a peppery way, but she was basically nice.

"Where is Daddy?" I asked.

"He's finishing up a round at the Worthington Golf Club," Uncle Allerton said. "But he'll be at the house when we get there."

Daddy was a geologist, but we knew he was out of work, as usual. He lived with his foster mother, Helen McCann, in her gorgeous summerhouse in Worthington.

"We're getting ready to go around some hills," Billy said.

I noticed Uncle Allerton honked his horn before he made a sharp turn. Up, up, and up. Very different than flat Florida. After Uncle

Allerton drove us up the long front driveway of Helen's house, Billy and I jumped out.

"Hello, kids," Daddy said.

I could see the red of his golf pants. "I like your pants," I said.

"You can't see," he said.

It felt like he'd driven a knife into my heart. I wanted to leave and go back home.

Billy helped me into the mudroom, where there was a nickel slot machine. Daddy gave us each a roll of nickels. Billy took my hand and showed me how to play. With my first nickel, I won five. I ended up winning twenty nickels, and Billy ended up winning thirty. We put them all in a cup to play again later.

That night Uncle Allerton picked up Daddy, Billy, and me. We couldn't understand why Daddy wasn't driving. Our uncle took us to his and Aunt Marjorie's summer house for dinner. I could sense right away that they lived in a much smaller house than Daddy and Helen. For *hors d'oeuvres* we had hard-boiled eggs with anchovies on top. I cannot stand anchovies. Aunt Marjorie served lamb with mint jelly. I continued to smell the whiskey Uncle Allerton and Daddy were drinking even at the dinner table.

"Peggy can't see," Daddy said right after we sat down.

I gripped the edge of the table, which was covered in a linen tablecloth. I felt destroyed.

"Well, I think she does really well," Aunt Marjorie said. "I think she is remarkable."

Billy kicked me under the table, which made me laugh a little. Aunt Marjorie had cut up my piece of lamb so I picked at it and the mint jelly. I don't really know what else was said. The only people there were Billy, me, Aunt Marjorie, Uncle Allerton, and Daddy.

The next day Billy and Daddy went to the Worthington Golf Club. Helen's nephew, Davy, had come to town so he went along. Billy and Daddy wanted to bet a milkshake on the round, but Davy had diabetes. He asked if they could all just bet a dollar on the game.

"I like his attitude," Daddy said later. "He acts positive about his handicap."

Did that mean I didn't? I wanted to go home. I pulled out a

strand of my hair and twirled it through my fingers.

The next day Daddy said Elizabeth, Helen's cook, was driving us into North Hampton to buy some legs of lamb and some beef roasts. He said Billy was staying behind to practice his golf. I sat in front with Elizabeth, and Daddy sat in back. We stopped at the butcher shop and then headed back to Worthington. I asked Daddy a question and he said, "Mmm?"

Then Daddy let out with a roar. When he fell silent, Elizabeth said, "He's having a seizure. We can't let him swallow his tongue." And she pulled to the side of the road.

She said, "He shouldn't drink. The doctors say drinking aggravates his seizures."

I said nothing until I walked into the mudroom and heard Billy on the slot machine. "I have to talk to you," I said.

"Let's go outside, Piglet."

We walked down the long driveway with me holding on to his arm. I hardly noticed the sound of the yard man on the power mower or the smell of newly cut grass.

"Daddy had a seizure in the car, Billy. We need to call Momma and go home. He roared like a lion."

"Really?" Billy said. He sounded surprised. Momma and Billy hardly ever sounded surprised. "Maybe that's why he's not driving," Billy continued.

"Billy," I said, "he has a handicap."

"You're right," Billy said. "Listen, there are at least ten phones in Helen's house. I'll go find one and call Momma on it."

After Billy called Momma, he came to my bedroom to report. Momma told him Daddy had epilepsy from falling off a horse as a teenager and hitting his head. She said she asked the doctor when she was pregnant with Billy if there was any genetic component, and he'd said that obviously there was not.

"But why didn't she tell us?" I asked.

"You know Momma doesn't tell us very much," Billy said.

Our plane was leaving in two days, and I was counting the minutes.

Chapter Eight

The following year, Momma was dating a guy named Clarence Haish. Billy said he was from one of the fine old Jacksonville families, and his father owned an investment firm. For some reason Clarence didn't work for his father's company. He was a civil engineer and had graduated from Georgia Tech. Billy said it looked like Clarence was going to take Momma to the River Club every Saturday night for dinner. The River Club was the most expensive club in Jacksonville.

One Saturday night Momma was going to the River Club with Clarence. One of her friends stopped by before she left and said she looked beautiful in pink. Billy had his girlfriend, Susan, over for pizza. The three of us young people ate some pizza at the dining room table, but then Billy and Susan holed up in the living room, and I could see under the door that they had turned out the lights. Later Momma and Clarence came back, and I heard them walk across the linoleum kitchen floor and into her bedroom. She had this room added on to the back of the house so she didn't have to sleep in the dining room any longer. Beany would not stop growling and barking at Clarence, so Momma in her high heels came right back out of her bedroom and said, "Go outside, Beany." Then I heard the kitchen screen door slam and assumed Momma had put Beany out.

Anyway, the room Momma had added on shared a wall with my bedroom. I could hear Momma and Clarence talking, but I couldn't hear what they said. About midnight I heard one of Clarence's heavy shoes drop on Momma's bedroom floor and wondered what was going on. Soon afterward, Momma and Clarence walked across the linoleum kitchen floor and toward the front door.

The next day I asked Momma why Clarence's shoe had dropped on the bedroom floor. She said he took his shoes off to stand on the bed and hang a picture on the wall. I hadn't heard any hammering. When Momma was in the bathroom, I went in her room and felt above the bed. No picture.

Momma mentioned that she had never liked Daddy's drinking, but of course Clarence drank as well. Momma said that if she married Clarence, we would have a lot of money. She said I could have a beautiful debut party and all the debut clothes I wanted. I remembered Momma hated being a debutante; she'd said it was that very year that she first started taking tranquilizers. Maybe it would be better to have more money. Momma had been born with a silver spoon and fallen into the middle class after her divorce. On the other hand, my wealthiest cousins had a child drown in the St. John's River. I reflected on various hardships.

***

I was spending the night at my grandmother's one day, and the telephone rang around midnight on my bedside table. It was Clarence, and he was looking for Momma. His words were slurred. "I think she's at home, Clarence," I said.

"She's not answering at home," he said. "Oh, shit." He hung up.

On the other side of the bed from the bedside table was the fireplace. I got out of bed and for some reason touched the mantelpiece. I liked fireplaces, and the conversation had not only awakened me, it had bothered me quite a bit. After a year of dating Clarence, Momma said she was breaking up with him because of his drinking. She said it was not worth putting up with the drinking for the money. Then Momma came home every day after school and got in bed. She smoked cigarettes and read *War and Peace.* She barely got Chef Boyardee and hotdogs and canned split pea soup on the table for dinner.

One night I asked her why she had cut the hotdogs up in the split pea soup. I told her I thought it would have been better to cook them separately.

"That would mean another damn pot to wash," she snapped.

I decided not to remind her that Billy and I did the dishes.

I heard Momma mention to a few friends that she was depressed.

One day, six months after Momma broke off their relationship, the phone rang. I was in the living room sitting sideways with my legs slung over the arm of a high-back chair. I jumped up and answered the phone, which was on the end table beside the sofa. It was Clarence. He said he had stopped drinking, and he wanted to ask me out to dinner. He said we would go to a steakhouse that didn't serve liquor. I asked if I could call him back. I thought about the whole thing. I had never particularly liked Clarence. Maybe I was jealous of him because he took up a lot of Momma's time. Beany barked her head off every time she saw him. But a steak dinner was, after all, a steak dinner. I asked Momma if I could go.

"Do you want to go, peach cake?"

"I guess so," I said.

"Then you can go. I saw Clarence's sister the other day, and she said he has stopped drinking."

So, I called Clarence back and accepted the invitation. I decided to wear my Easter dress, which I knew was blue linen with a white linen collar. I had some high-heeled white shoes and a white purse. I hoped the shoes and purse were free of spots. Momma didn't notice things like that.

At 6:30 Saturday night the doorbell rang. I knew it must be Clarence. Beany was barking and barking. I had to push her away from the door so I could squeeze out onto the porch.

"You look pretty tonight," Clarence said, and he put my arm through his. I felt good so far.

We walked down our five front steps. There were no railings. I had three thoughts: Clarence did not smell like liquor; Billy had told me once that Clarence looked like Yul Brynner, and it was hot outside.

My heart started beating quickly. I wasn't sure if I should go to dinner with Clarence by myself. Momma had said to let her know when I got home. I knew she wouldn't ask me any questions. She just didn't want to see Clarence. I hadn't told my grandmother I was going out to dinner with Clarence, and I was pretty sure my mother hadn't either. Grandmomma would have been beside herself. She'd liked Clarence fine until Momma broke up with him. Then she pointed out that Clarence didn't get along with his father, and said that was why he didn't work with his father and that he probably just didn't get along with people. She said she'd had to correct a few people who said Clarence broke up with Momma. She said she'd told them it was entirely the other way around.

Clarence helped me into his Cadillac, which was a lot more comfortable than Momma's old Rambler. I heard him get in on his side and start the engine.

"What color is your car?" I asked.

"White with a black interior," he said, and turned on the radio. "I invited my nieces who are your age to go with us to dinner, but my sister said they couldn't go tonight."

Frank Sinatra sang forth. We drove to the end of my street and turned right and drove along what I knew was Willow Branch Avenue with the park and the wooden bridge.

At the steakhouse we sat in a booth. The cushion was hard. I figured anyone who saw me would notice my blind, disfigured eyes. Grandmomma kept saying I really needed a new prosthesis for my right eye. The restaurant was not really dark. The three-man band played sixties music.

"How is your mother?" Clarence asked.

"Oh, fine," I said.

"She is beautiful," Clarence said.

Our steaks came. I asked Clarence to cut mine up, and he did. Someone dropped a plate, and I heard it shatter into pieces. "Why did the waiter drop that plate?" Clarence said. He sounded agitated.

"I don't know," I said. "I think they just drop them sometimes."

"But why break a plate?" Clarence asked.

"I'm sure it was an accident," I said, wondering what the big deal was. "You've been horseback riding?" I asked because Clarence used to take Momma horseback riding.

"No," Clarence said and fell silent. He muttered something under his breath about the plate breaking.

When we left, I tried to hold on to Clarence's arm above the elbow but he insisted on linking my arm through his. On the way home, Clarence stopped the car and said we were at a railroad crossing. I sure hoped we weren't parked over the track. "I wish you could see that man in the orange shirt walking down the track," he said. He laughed and then he kept on laughing. I couldn't figure out why, and I felt very uncomfortable.

When we walked up the front steps of my front porch, Beany started barking. When I opened the door, Beany became frantic.

"Good night and thanks," I said loudly and squeezed myself in. I calmed Beany down. It would be appropriate to write Clarence a thank-you note. I went back to speak to Momma.

"Did you have a good time?" she asked.

"It was okay," I said. "But when a waiter drops a plate and breaks it, don't you think it was an accident?"

"Sure," Momma said between puffs on her cigarette. "Listen, you should get *Tess of the d'Urbervilles* on a talking-book record. It's really good. By the way, can you make me a cup of coffee?"

"Okay," I said. I made my way into the kitchen and filled a pot partway with water from the sink. Placing it on a burner, I turned the knob to high. I found the jar of coffee and shook it to make sure there were crystals inside. I located a cup and saucer, which I knew were Momma's red-and-white Vista China pattern. When I heard the water boil, I poured some into the cup until it met the bottom of my index finger. It burned momentarily but the sensation went away. I measured out a teaspoon of coffee crystals and stirred them into the hot water. Where was Beany? I sure didn't want to trip over her. Assuming she was still in the living room, I carefully carried the cup and saucer back to my mother, who was sitting in bed.

"You're a fine girl," Momma said. "This is just what I wanted."

***

Once in a while Momma watched and I listened to the 6:00 news. Three days after I had gone to dinner with Clarence, she turned on the black-and-white TV in the living room. The announcer said, "The son of a very prominent Jacksonville citizen was arrested for murdering his aunt. Clarence Haish Jr., son of investment-firm owner Clarence Haish Sr., was arrested this afternoon at the home of his aunt for murdering her. He called the police to say he had shot and killed her with a shotgun."

"Clarence is in handcuffs!" Momma exclaimed in surprise.

The phone started ringing. My mind raced. Why did Clarence shoot his aunt? I was glad he hadn't shot me. He sure hadn't seemed violent. I thought about the strange comments he'd made about the waiter breaking the plate and the man walking down the railroad track.

I later learned that Momma and Clarence had both been seeing the same psychiatrist. Clarence had been diagnosed with paranoid schizophrenia, and he apparently also sometimes spoke of wanting to harm others, but the psychiatrist had not revealed Clarence's illness to Momma.

Today a psychiatrist would have "the duty to warn," due to the Tarasoff Decision. In 1969, a university student named Prosenjit Poddar told a campus psychologist that he wanted to kill his former girlfriend, Tatiana Tarasoff. The psychologist and his supervisor notified campus police but not the girl or her family. Poddar ultimately killed Tarasoff with a kitchen knife. A few years later, in a suit her parents had brought against the doctors and the university, a judge ruled that the duty to warn a third party who was being threatened by a patient outweighed the patient's right to confidentiality. The patient's doctor had a "duty to warn" the person who was being threatened.

Clarence had murdered his father's sister, but his father felt he had to hire a lawyer to defend his son. The upshot of it all was that Mr. Haish Sr. had the money to keep Clarence out of jail. Clarence ended up having to spend the rest of his life in a psychiatric hospital in Tampa. If he had walked out of the hospital, he would have had to stand trial for murder.

Momma didn't say much about Clarence and that situation. She said she was awfully glad Clarence hadn't shot me. But then Clarence's story was moved to Momma's list of taboo topics, and we never talked about it again. I gave Beany a really big hug for being so perceptive.

***

In the tenth grade, I attended Jacksonville Episcopal High School. All my classes were very challenging, and I loved each and every one, except geometry.

A fun thing I got to do was wear a miniskirt every day. One skirt was described to me as looking like a Chagall painting. The school had a rule that girls couldn't wear dresses or skirts more than two inches above the knee, but I never got in trouble for my miniskirts which came to ten inches above the knee. The other girls didn't like that at all. The teachers and administrators probably gave me a pass because I was blind. Oh, that word—"blind."

Throughout high school, my swollen right eye with the hernia bothered me greatly. I didn't see why Dr. K failed to enucleate the eye so that a new prosthesis could fit much better. But now I was scared of Dr.

K. Momma never said a thing about the prosthesis and the swollen eye, but she was an auditory, not a visual person. Still, I was very angry with her. Grandmomma commented on it often. I really suffered over the eye. When I felt it, it protruded so far out of my face. And yearbook pictures were a nightmare. Some of my classmates commented on how big my right eye looked in the photos.

"Why, Momma, why?" I wanted to cry out. "High school is such an important time for appearance."

One day in tenth grade one day I touched a column next to the entrance of the high school and liked the smooth feel of the bricks. I listened for the sound of Mrs. Valentine's car. Mrs. Valentine was picking me up for my cane-traveling lesson. She was new to the field of cane travel, but I liked her, and I was learning a lot.

I heard Mrs. Valentine's quiet engine as she stopped her car in front of me. As I climbed in, she said, "I brought you a cheeseburger and fries."

"Yum," I said, and dived right in.

We drove to the bus stop on Park Street a few blocks from my house. Mrs. Valentine loaned me a white cane. So far, I hadn't wanted to walk around school with one, and I could get around the high school based solely on memory. Mrs. Valentine and I rode the bus to a bus stop near J.C. Penney's. When we got off the bus, we had to cross Bay Street at the intersection of Broad Street to reach the store. Mrs. Valentine explained that there was a traffic light here, but that, since I couldn't see it, I would have to listen to the traffic. She said not to go by the sound of traffic stopping on Bay, but instead, to listen for the sound of traffic starting up on Broad, parallel to our direction of travel. When I heard that sound, I could cross Bay. I should use my white cane. She also said that the side of Penney's facing me was painted red—a good, and rare, visual cue. We practiced crossing at the intersection and walking up to Penney's several times, but we didn't work on going inside.

We headed back to the bus stop and got off at Park Street. Once we were back in the car, I asked Mrs. Valentine if we could drop the white cane off at my house. I wanted one there but not at school. I didn't use the white cane in my neighborhood until that Saturday, when I told Momma I was going to take the bus downtown. She said that would be fine. She was in bed, reading *Great Expectations*.

On the way to the bus stop, I didn't need the cane, so I twirled it through my fingers like a baton. I found the bus stop at the corner of Park and McDuff and felt for the bench, then sat down and waited for the roar of the bus and the smell of the fumes. When the bus stopped and the door cranked open, I put my white cane forward and asked if this was Bus 20, going to town.

"Yes, sweetie," the male bus driver said.

"Can I sit by the door across from you?" I asked, as I climbed onto the bus, gripping my cane in my right hand.

"Someone is already sitting there," the driver said. "But you can sit right in back of me. Where are you going?"

"Broad and Bay," I said. I found the pole next to the driver's seat, located the empty seat behind him, sat down and braced the cane. Then I remembered, "Can I hand you the fare?"

"I got it," the driver said. I wondered what he thought of the appearance of my eyes.

"She's blind," someone whispered.

That word really bothered me. It made me feel depressed, angry, helpless and isolated. I gritted my teeth and sat silently as the bus moved toward town.

"Have you always been blind?" the driver's voice floated back at me. I didn't answer. I didn't want to talk about it. I tried to think of something pleasant. But before I could, the driver said, "We're at Broad and Bay."

When I stood up someone whispered, "The blind girl is getting off here."

"Do you want me to help you off?" the driver asked.

"It's okay," I said. Holding my cane slightly in front of me, I made my way down the steps to the sidewalk. I successfully crossed Bay Street at the intersection with Broad. As soon as the parallel traffic started on Broad, I stepped out into Bay and walked beside the sound of parallel traffic. Then I looked for the red wall of Penney's. Mrs. Valentine had not taught me how to go through the glass doors of the department store and inside on my own, but I would figure it out.

I listened for people's voices increasing in volume as they pushed their way out through the glass doors. My fear was that a sighted person might hold the door for me but not realize he or she should tell me the door was now open. I hoped I could simply feel along the smooth glass and find the handle, which was what happened. I opened the door and triumphantly stepped into Penney's.

"Where do you want to go?" someone nearby yelled at me. Sometimes people thought I was also deaf and maybe mentally deficient.

"The lingerie department," I replied in an even tone.

The person grabbed my arm and immediately pushed me into a rack of brand-new clothes.

"Hold on a minute," I said. "Please let me hang on to your arm just above the elbow. This is the way we ask sighted people to guide us."

The woman understood. We walked along with my hand on her arm slightly above her elbow.

"Here we are," my guide said.

"What do you want?" another woman asked, in a condescending voice. It sounded like she was behind a counter.

"Five pair of size-five underwear," I said.

"Can you see the colors?" the same woman asked, in a somewhat friendlier tone.

I had my hand on the smooth glass counter now, and felt more oriented. I was on my side of it, and the saleswoman was on her side. "No, I can't," I said.

"What happened to your eyes?" the woman asked.

"I don't know," I said.

"Well, here's the underwear," the woman said. A bag crinkled as she set it on the counter. "That will be $5.15."

I had a five-dollar bill folded in a special way in my wallet, and I found a dime and a nickel by feel. I handed the money toward her.

"Do you need to go somewhere else in the store?" she asked.

"To the front door, please," I said. "Let me hold on to your arm just above the elbow."

I took her elbow and she walked me between the racks. I took a last, deep breath of the new-clothes scent. I could see the outside light. I remembered I had pulled the door toward me coming in, so I would push it outward to exit.

"I feel so sorry for her," I heard my saleswoman whisper.

"I can make it from here," I said. I broke away and walked toward the light. I found the glass door and pushed. I knew I should tap my white cane in front of me when walking to the bus stop, but I just held it in my hand as I walked to the corner of Broad and Bay. It was not until I began to cross Bay that I began to tap my cane.

Chapter Nine

Grandmomma, Momma, and I were eating dessert in Grandmomma's dining room. "Aren't you going to eat your Lady Baltimore cake?" Grandmomma said.

"I don't know," Momma said, and I heard her take a sip of coffee and the sound of the China cup being placed in the saucer.

"Mary Jean, sit up straight. You will ruin your posture," said Grandmomma. "I pray you will find a nice husband."

"There just aren't enough nice men to go around," Momma said.

"I have to go home and pay bills. I need to call a carpenter to repair two boards that are rotting on my front porch. And I need him to replace two more that are rotting around my toilet. Actually, the toilet isn't working very well so I need to call a plumber."

The last time a plumber had come to our house, I was a teenager, but Momma made me stay with her in the living room.

"By the way, where is Beany?" Grandmomma asked

"I left her in the house with the air conditioner on," Momma said. "She's probably sleeping on my good white sofa. The cat threw up on the dining room table yesterday, and I scrubbed the table with BAB-O. Now the table has light spots, and the wood grain looks strange."

"Let me read you this newspaper article from November 21, 1946," Grandmomma said. "'Mrs. Herbert Lamson has tea feting daughter in Riverside Avenue home.'"

"The year I made my debut, I started taking tranquilizers."

Grandmomma ignored her and continued, "'The tea was given at the home of Mrs. Lamson yesterday afternoon between the hours of 4 and 6 o'clock. It was given by Mrs. Lamson in honor of her daughter, Miss Mary Jean Lamson.'"

"Hey, Grandmomma," I said. "I went downtown the other day and went to Penney's and bought some underwear."

"I don't want you taking the bus from home to town. You are handicapped."

"I think it's all right if she does," Momma said.

"No, it is not," Grandmomma said.

"Excuse me for a minute," Momma said, and left the room.

I said, "I think you upset Momma."

"Take your hands out of your mouth, Peggy. You're pulling it out of shape. You'll ruin it. I'll never understand your mother. Now tell me what happened at school today."

"Well, after lunch I was trying to find a column with a trash can beside it. I wanted to throw out a carton of iced tea. I looked for a shadow beside a column and saw one. My carton was still about half full. I threw it and somebody began to laugh. It was a boy. I said 'I'm sorry, I thought you were the garbage can.' I could hear the tea dripping onto the sidewalk, but he was nice about it."

"What was his name?" Grandmomma laughed.

"I don't know."

"Come on back in, Mary Jean," Grandmomma called. Momma walked in and sat down. She took a sip of her coffee and set it back in the saucer.

"This Lady Baltimore cake is delicious," Grandmomma said, and her fork rang against her China plate. "Don't you want to eat your cake, Mary Jean?"

"I don't know," Momma said. "Like I said, I have to go home and pay the bills. I have to do something about the grass in my front and back yards. Grass never grows there."

"Oh—where was I in the clipping?" Grandmomma asked. "Here. 'An antique tureen holding yellow and gold chrysanthemums was used in decorating the hall. The living room was decorated with fall blossoms and greens. The dining-room table was overlaid with a white organdy cloth appliqued with linen and was centered by a gold China compote flanked by brass candelabra holding ivory tapers. At either end, the coffee and tea services were placed.'"

"Mother, I hated that party."

"'Mrs. Lamson and her debutante daughter received their guests in the living room in front of the bay window, where a brass bowl held gold and yellow chrysanthemums.'"

"I don't know why you didn't enjoy your debut year, Mary Jean. Your father and I broke our backs to buy beautiful dresses."

"I hated the parties, and I broke up with Theodore that summer. We had been dating two years, since we were seniors in high school. I loved his wild driving and his late-night style."

"Mother, I'm going home." Her voice turned my way. "Do you want to go home?"

"I'll stay and talk to Clara for a little while. I can probably walk home with my cane."

"No," Grandmomma said. "I will take you home when I take Clara. Mary Jean, I'm going to call the beauty parlor and make an appointment for you to get your hair done. Listen to this: 'Miss Lamson was gowned in gold with short sleeves and a scalloped neckline and a fitted bodice and a full skirt. Long satin gloves were worn, and she carried a bird-of-paradise bouquet.'"

"Mother, I need to go home. I'm depressed. In addition to everything else, I need to have the right passenger door of my car repaired."

"What is the matter with you, Mary Jean? Look at all I do. I take the children to the doctor and the dentist and to Scouts and to piano lessons and to cello lessons, and I take the dog to the vet. And I pay your Colonial Dames dues and your Junior League dues."

"I resigned from the Junior League once, and I'm about to resign again," Momma said.

"Don't you dare."

Momma pushed back her chair and walked to the front door.

"I'm going to talk to Clara," I said.

The kitchen was hot. Clara said "Hello, darlin'," and I heard the stool she pushed toward me across the floor.

"I'm doing dishes," Clara said, as the water splashed on the newspaper in front of the sink.

"Can you tell me about when I was little, Clara?"

"Well, darlin'," Clara said. "The first time I came to see y'all, I took the train—the Silver Meteor—from Jacksonville to Fort Worth. You were four months old, and Billy was two years old. You were an ugly baby. All bald-headed, as I have told you. Billy was pretty and laughing down. He loved fried chicken. I still had some from my lunch on the train, and I gave him a drumstick. I stayed for two weeks with your mother. It was so different in Fort Worth from Jacksonville. There were lots of beautiful houses like Jacksonville, but there were no trees. I came back on the Silver Meteor.

"You were about one when your daddy got a job in Midland, and your family moved there. Doctors said you couldn't live there because of the dust, so you came to live in Jacksonville with your grandmother and grandfather and me until you were two. Then your parents moved to Houston, and you went out there with them.

"The next time I saw you was in New York. That was a bad time. I took the Silver Meteor, and your grandfather fixed it so I could take a taxi straight to the hotel. He paid for the taxi, and he paid for your mother and you and me to stay in the hotel. It was a nice hotel. It was eighteen dollars a day.

"Your mother was so happy to see me. I took you to the hospital every day for your eye, and your mother stayed back at the hotel. She didn't go far. That was life, darlin'; we couldn't help it. That was life."

"I wish I could see, Clara."

"I know it darlin', but God is able." Clara came over, and I stood up, and she held me tight. If I could have cried, I would've cried right then.

***

Once in a while my grandmother took me to Clara's house to spend the afternoon on Clara's day off. On one such day I needed to go because I was writing a paper about Clara for English class. On this particular day she told me a story about a snake.

"Course, it could have been there all night," Clara began. "This

God is so good to me. I got up that morning and raised the shade as usual. I jumped back. I saw this black snake curled up in the window. So, I looked at him, and he didn't move. So, I didn't get scared. We had snakes on Daddy's farm, and I thought he was a harmless snake, but I wasn't taking any chances. I turned around and walked over to the front. I looked at the Salvation Army, and I was going to go over there. So, I walked down my front steps, and a man was walking by from across town. So, I said, 'Come here now. I'm in distress. There is a snake in my window.'"

"He said, 'I'm going to look for a job.'"

"So I said, 'I'll give you something.'"

"So, he came, and we looked at the snake, and it never moved. So the man said, 'Do you have a shovel?'"

"And I said, there's one in the corner. I told him I wanted to go out because I didn't want to be there."

Clara took a breath.

"So, then I walked out, and I think he put the shovel on him because he knocked the whole screen out and blood was on the shovel. I think he was a harmless snake, but if he wasn't, he could have come in the window by my head, and I could have died. When the man knocked the snake out, he opened the back door and looked out there and the snake was lying on the other side. So, I asked him what to do now. He said to get some hot water. We threw the hot water over that side. And then the man asked if I had some turpentine. Snakes hate turpentine. So, we poured turpentine on him. Then I had to get Robert to come fix my screen. I just recently started sleeping with my head under that window again.

"I thought that snake sure was dead after being hit by a shovel, thrown out a window, and having hot water and turpentine poured on him."

I wondered what a snake looked like. I pictured everything by feel. I had felt a stuffed snake but would probably be afraid of a live one.

"So, you grew up on a farm, right Clara?"

"Yes."

"What did your father raise on his farm at Windfield besides cotton and tobacco?"

Clara said, "Corn, tomatoes, sweet potatoes, and peanuts."

"What did you do to help around the farm?"

"I picked string beans and corn and tomatoes and cotton and tobacco and peanuts. And cooked things like string beans and corn. I cooked since I was eight years old."

"Where did you go to school, Clara?"

"I went to school in Columbia County. I liked school but did not get through the fifth grade."

"What's your favorite color?" I asked.

"Blue and green."

"What is your favorite food?"

"Sweet potatoes, collard greens, shrimp pilau, cauliflower, and eggplant."

"What's your favorite smell?" I asked.

"Roses."

"What do you like the feel of?"

"Velvet."

"What sounds do you like?"

"The sound of a bell is beautiful."

"What do you like to look at in nature?"

"I like to watch the birds play and talk and whistle."

"If you had one wish, what would it be?"

"I would wish for good health."

"If you had one statement about God, what would it be?"

"God is good."

"Are there any songs you like to sing besides 'East Side West Side' and 'Lord, I Ain't No Stranjuh Now?'"

Clara said, "Jesus, Keep Me Near the Cross."

"Which word do you like better: think or feel?"

Clara said, "I like both of them."

"What is the happiest time or moment in your life?"

"The happiest time is now. Just as well to be."

"What would you tell me about Willie?"

"I was married to Willie for 22 years. He worked at a filling station. And then he was a chauffeur for the Myerheims. They lived across the street from your grandparents in Jacksonville. Then they moved to St. Petersburg, and Willie went with them. He sent for me so we could get married. I took the Greyhound bus to St. Petersburg, and we were married by the Justice of the Peace. Then Willie got a job back in Jacksonville, and I kept working for your grandparents. But you can't brag on men. They ain't much.

"A few years ago, James moved in with me as a boarder. We bought a refrigerator together, and he kept stocking it with beer. I barely had enough room for the food I fixed for him and he paid me for. He didn't have anything to do. He had worked at Rexall Drugs for 41 years and then retired. All he did here was drink beer."

"Hey Clara, I have to ask you something. Did my great grandmother go to Milledgeville?"

"She did."

This intrigued me. The hospital in Milledgeville, Georgia, was for mentally ill people. I thought very mentally ill.

I felt so good around Clara. It seemed like my blindness didn't matter to her. I had asked her so many questions about her life, because I was writing my next English paper about her. I wanted to surprise her by reading her the Braille copy when I finished it.

**

In high school, I studied all the time. I won quite a few scholastic awards, but I had few friends. I felt lonely, and envied the popular students. In May of my senior year, I had spring fever. I was taking third-year Latin from Mr. King, and we were translating Cicero. He assigned 100 lines a night for us to translate. One night I listened to the *Andy Griffith Show* and *Green Acres* instead of doing my Latin homework. Naturally, the next day in class, Mr. King called on me to recite the translated lines.

I was at a loss for words. My classmate Mary, who sat across from me, tried to whisper the translation to me, but Mr. King told her to stop talking.

"Mr. King, I'm sorry, but I just didn't have time to do my Latin homework last night."

I had really had it with homework. I didn't do it that night either. I played with Beany, Wicky the cat, and Sugar the rabbit. Of course, Mr. King called on me the next day, and again, I didn't know the lines. The other students in the class chuckled because I had never behaved in such an irresponsible way. And then, for the third night in a row, I didn't do my homework. The next morning, Mr. King called on me yet again. He always remained calm.

At the end of the semester, surprisingly, I ended up with an A-minus in Latin, probably because I'd made 105 on every test. At high school graduation in June of 1971, in addition to receiving academic awards, I received an award for excellence of character.

"You're a character, all right," Billy said.

I just laughed.

I was on my way to Wheaton College, near Boston in the fall. We had college counselors at Episcopal, and they nudged us toward the Northeast. I was accepted to colleges in the South and the North. The two that admitted me in the Northeast were Smith and Wheaton. Although Smith was more prestigious, I decided not to go there, because my father was living 24 miles from the campus. He made me very nervous. So, I was going to Wheaton, which was 150 miles from his house.

***

I went to Wheaton in the fall of 1971. Momma didn't seem to have any qualms about my flying off to Boston by myself, and taking a taxi to Wheaton. She shipped me my trunk.

I had taken out my prosthesis and understood my right eye appeared as white with red lines. Momma didn't seem at all concerned about sending me off to college that way. She only let me buy a few winter outfits, and it was too warm to wear them at first. I just wore jeans and a Wheaton t-shirt.

Wheaton housing assigned me to a single room, which I didn't understand. Why not a roommate like the other freshman girls? I obtained my books in Braille or on tape, and dove into studying. Wheaton made a private library room available to me. I spent a great deal of time there. That way my tapes, which played out loud, would not annoy other students. I felt very isolated.

My creative writing professor approved of the title of my first paper: "How Great Independence." In it, I detailed my trip alone on the bus to Penney's and back for the first time.

At the college, I learned the campus fairly quickly. I requested a psychologist, and was assigned to a Dr. Wright. He was a very sympathetic old man who told me he was bow-legged and, therefore, he had some sense of disfigurement.

The girls I met asked me why I spent so much time at the library. I explained that making good grades was extremely important to me. They said that studying was important to them, but they said they also liked to socialize. They acted like I was weird, whispering within earshot, "There she goes to the library again."

For the second paper for my creative writing class, professor approval of the title was not required. I wrote about my hostility toward blindness. The professor, Mrs. Shaw, said she was not going to grade the paper. She said there were six papers to be written for the class, and she would just grade me on five. I didn't understand at all. Why was my paper on independence graded, and my paper on hostility toward blindness not graded? A punching bag named Mrs. Shaw seemed like a good idea.

***

I did have one fun weekend in the great dreary fall. Susie Smith, who lived on my floor of the dorm, asked me home to Boston for the weekend. Susie was very sweet, but she had a bad stutter. People said she was very cute and had a beautiful complexion. For the first time in my life, my skin was breaking out.

So, on a cold, late October day, Susie took me to her dad's apartment in Boston. Her parents were divorced, and she didn't get along with her mother. Susie had a boyfriend named John, and he set me up with a couple of blind dates. A fun thing to do! On Friday night we went to Boston College. I had a date with a guy named Christopher. He said everyone in the world was a derelict, a deviant, or a degenerate.

The next night I had a date with Larry. Susie, John, Larry and I went to a Halloween party. Susie put together a costume for me: a Hawaiian dancer. She placed artificial flowers on me, and I wore a grass paper skirt. She made a tight-fitting satin blouse for me to wear as well. Susie went as a flapper, and her boyfriend, John, went as a clown. My date Larry went as a mummy wrapped in toilet paper, and we wondered if his costume, or my grass paper skirt would fall apart first.

These were the only two dates I had in my three semesters at Wheaton. Many of the girls dated guys from Brown which was only 15 miles away. I blamed the blindness and the disfigurement and felt terrible about my situation. Was suicide an option?

Toward the end of Fall Semester, I was walking across campus on a snowy grey day. It seemed as if the sun never shone. Someone spoke, and I stopped. I realized it was Mrs. Shaw, the English professor.

"How are you, Peggy?"

"Fine, thanks," I said, immediately remembering my paper on hostility toward blindness, which she never graded.

"You wrote a number of good papers," she said. "The best one was on independence: traveling on the bus from your home to downtown Jacksonville and back. It was amazing."

I looked in her direction as best I could. "I will not be defeated," I said defiantly. And I walked away as quickly as possible.

"I know you won't," she called after me.

***

At Christmas I went home to sunny Florida for a month. Disappointment and anger set in. Momma had gone to Germany for two weeks to see Billy, who was taking his junior year abroad.

Grandmomma kept saying, "We need to do something about your complexion. And we must do something about your right eye. It doesn't look natural."

Depression deepened, and my head dropped down. My good grades hardly mattered to me.

Momma did come back for the last two weeks of my vacation. She said she was proud of me for going to Wheaton. Adding to my depression however, was that I had to read the book *The Plague*, by Camus, for my upcoming English class.

***

Before summer, I was invited to make my debut.

Grandmomma called and said, "Peggy, it would be wonderful for you to make your debut."

The socially prominent and beautiful girls in my age group who would certainly be asked to make their debuts came to mind. To go to parties with them and my disfigured eyes made me feel sick.

Momma called and said, "Don't make your debut. Each debutante has to give one big party, and I don't have the money to give you one."

"That's okay, Momma. I'm going to decline my debut."

***

I hated spring semester at Wheaton. All I did was study. When I touched my swollen right eye, I felt revolted.

Surprisingly, the summer of 1972 had some good happenings. Doctor K enucleated my right eye. That made it far less swollen. Late in the summer I was able to get a somewhat better prosthesis. Not perfect but an improvement.

In the meantime, my eyes were still fairly disfigured.

However, I gritted my teeth, and I attended many of the lavish debut parties. Usually, a guy named Jimmy from one of the fine old families escorted me. We had a lot of fun, and he always complimented me on my evening gowns. We went to dances at country clubs, and came home at 4:00 am. Momma was sound asleep. She never worried about what time Billy or I got home. She was a laissez-faire parent.

I went back to Wheaton in the fall with dread. I told Momma I might have to transfer to Florida State sometime. She said I should do whatever I wanted to do.

In the fall of 1972 I lived in a single room attached to a double room. My roommates in the double room were worried about me. I spent all my time at the library.

During that fall, a new English professor, Mrs. Riggio, invited me home to Boston for the weekend. She and her husband and I went to see the movie *The Godfather*. I couldn't believe all the red I saw in the movie. Mrs. Riggio said it was blood.

By Thanksgiving, Momma said she had applied for me to attend Florida State, in case I might want to go in January of 1973. It was very surprising for Momma to act on my behalf, but I couldn't wait to get back to the sunny South.

So, I went back to Wheaton for a few weeks and finished up Fall Semester right before Christmas. Daddy came over to Wheaton and helped me pack up my things and ship my trunk to Jacksonville. We had a brief but okay visit.

***

Prior to beginning winter quarter at Florida State in January of 1973, I flew to Germany to spend a week with my brother.

Billy was working in a post office there. He had returned to Germany after graduating from Johns Hopkins in December, 1972. He had fallen in love with Germany during his junior year abroad there, and wanted to spend additional time in the country after graduation.

My mother took me to the Jacksonville airport on January 2nd. She gave me a big hug and said she knew I would be just fine. I took a deep breath of her Arpege perfume before I was escorted onto the plane. We flew to Miami, and then a gate agent helped me to my connecting flight to London. Travel always gave me the feeling I needed a shower, but there was no help for it. Multiplying numbers in my head gave me something to do to entertain myself during the long flight from Miami to London. Two times two is four. Four times two is eight. Eight times two is sixteen. Sixteen times two is thirty-two. Thirty-two times two is sixty-four. Sixty-four times two is one-twenty-eight and so on.

I liked to get as high as 1,024 times two equals 2,048. When I got bored with math, I tried to sleep, but to no avail.

My plane from Miami to London arrived late in London. The agent said he would Telex an agent in Frankfurt, asking him to let my brother know I had missed my connection and would be late. However, Billy never got the message. He met my scheduled flight, and then met the next four coming from London to Frankfurt. He told me later he called up mother in Jacksonville and asked her if I had left Jacksonville yet. Mother said I had left hours earlier, but she was sure I would be fine.

I didn't make it on to any of the three flights from London to Frankfurt after missing my scheduled one. They were all booked. I made it on to the fourth flight. Billy actually met my flight. However, at that time, disabled people in the U.S. got off flights first. But in Europe they got off last. So, when I wasn't one of the first fifteen people off that flight, Billy left.

When I stepped into the Frankfurt airport, my brother wasn't there. I was exhausted and afraid. Everyone was talking in German, but finally an agent speaking in English spoke to me. I asked him to page my brother, and he said they only paged outgoing passengers.

At that point, I said my brother was the only person I knew on the continent of Europe, and to please page him. The agent did so, referring to me as "Ein kind Margaret Paul..." I was distressed, because I was twenty years old.

My brother finally found me, and we fell into each other's arms. We rushed to call our mother in Jacksonville.

"I knew you would make it," she said. "I really wasn't very worried."

On my trip abroad, my brother and I had the most interesting time when we went to Paris for a few days. We climbed the Eiffel Tower, visited Pere Lachaise Cemetery to visit the grave of Oscar Wilde (Billy's favorite author at that time), and toured Notre Dame. I stood on the spot there where Joan of Arc had stood. I rejoiced in the moment, and I will never forget her birth and death dates. She was born in 1412 and died in 1431.

***

When I returned to Florida State to begin Winter Quarter, things went okay. The roommates were all right; the readers were good, and my grades were great. Best of all, the sun shone most of the time. Also, I swam laps in the university pool every day.

The following year, 1974, I fell into a depression over my blindness. I was also unhappy that I never had a date.

One day, I decided to run away. I packed a grocery bag with a few clothes, some apples, some bananas, and a jar of peanut butter. I took a taxi from my dorm to the Greyhound bus station and bought a ticket to Atlanta. I didn't know anyone in Atlanta. I rode the bus there and then took a taxi to a bar, where I met several men including one named George. After we talked a while in the bar, I decided to leave with him. George had told me he worked as a taxi driver.

George held the passenger door of his taxi open, and I got in, dragging my white cane and grocery bag with me. I heard him open the driver's-side door and then his blue jeans sliding across the driver's seat.

"What is that smell?" I asked.

"Air freshener," he said. "I spray it in here when the drunks throw up."

"Did I tell you all the towns I went through on the Greyhound?" I asked.

"Name the towns," he said.

"From Tallahassee we went to Moultrie, and then to Tifton, and then to Ashburn, and then to Cordele, and then to Perry, and then to Macon, and then to Barnesville, and then to Griffin, and then to Jonesboro, and then to East Point, and finally to Atlanta."

"Why did you run away from college?" George asked.

"Because I am blind, and I want to die. I want to be buried with all our relatives in our plot in Evergreen Cemetery."

"You want to die because you're blind?"

"Yes. I'm depressed. And when I'm buried, I wonder if I'll find out that worms have evolved far enough to be choosy. Where they only want to eat dead sighted eyes."

"That is crazy," George said. "Listen, my roommate Harry and I are living in a house on Georgia Avenue. We hear the planes coming and going. We're real close to the airport."

"Did you go to college, George?" I asked, feeling a little uneasy.

"Yeah. Three years at Penn State. I hated college. You trot around to all your little classes."

"What do you do besides drive a cab?" I asked.

"I'm a bouncer in a bar. I'm six-foot six and weigh 250 pounds. By the way, what's in that grocery bag?"

"Apples, bananas, and a jar of peanut butter. Oh, and a body shirt to wear tomorrow. I could wear these jeans again. I never wear underwear."

"I didn't know you were blind in the bar at first," George said. "I thought you were barbed out. Did any other guys talk to you?"

"Yeah. A white guy and a black guy. The white guy said he was a carpenter and that he could make me happy if I went home with him. The black guy said he had never had a white lady. He said he'd just been fired from a school in Statesboro for talking to a white teacher."

I looked out the window at the streetlights.

"Did you like that Scotch and water you were drinking?" George asked.

"It was my first alcoholic drink, and it was bitter. I still drink

Shirley Temples at the Yacht Club in Jacksonville," I replied.

I thought about the linen tablecloths and linen napkins and sterling-silver place settings in the Yacht Club dining room. We always went out on the dock after dinner. It would be dark, and I'd listen to the waves of the St. John's River. I heard something rolling around on the cab floor.

"What was that?" I asked.

"It's a cue ball I stole from a pool hall," George said. "You can have it."

The hard ball hit my foot, and I picked it up off the cab floor. I put it in my grocery bag.

"George, what time is it?"

"Midnight."

I heard an airplane overhead. "Are we at your house?" I asked.

"Yes," George said. I felt him parallel-park the cab.

"I think you are a far-out chick," George said.

I started to ask if I could use the phone inside to call my brother. I didn't want to talk to my mother. But on second thought, I didn't want to call anybody.

"Listen, Peggy, there are lots of steps to the front door. I'll come get you." I got out with my white cane and grocery bag in hand and stood still. I felt for George's elbow on his huge arm. I placed my hand just above his elbow so he could guide me.

"I got my Harley motorcycle out here," he said. "I used to ride with a gang. Now ten steps up."

"A gang?" I said, and shivered. "Did you ever kill anyone?"

"One time we beat up a loner. I think we killed him. Let me unlock the door. I got guns above my couch, but you can't fool around with them."

We stepped inside onto a thin rug. George put my hand on the end of the couch. The material felt rough. I found a cushion and carefully sat down next to the arm of the couch.

"I'm going to fix us a cheese sandwich and a glass of milk," George said.

"George, do you think my eyes look okay?"

"They look all right. Quit talking about being blind. I'm tired of it," he said, and he lumbered out of the room.

I thought about Momma. "You are a fine, pretty girl, and lots of men will want to go out with you," she always said.

I asked her once if I would be better-looking if my eyes looked normal. Her voice quavered, and she said yes. *The guns! The wall behind the couch.* I stood up. Maybe I had time to shoot myself.

"Oh no you don't!" George said. "The cops have already been out here twice for dope. Sit down. You have your cheese sandwich. And I'm putting a glass of milk on a magazine on the table to your right. The magazine is called *Easy Rider*. It is all about nice tits, nice bikes, and nice asses. You have a nice ass. You want to ball later?"

"Probably not," I said. I took a bite of my sandwich.

George came back with his plate and sat down next to me on the couch. His huge thigh touched mine. I heard a thud overhead.

"What was that?" I asked.

"Cathy and Kevin live up there. Cathy was a whore before. That's not Kevin's kid. Cathy used to look like a floozy. Greasy black wig and makeup. I taught her how to do her own makeup and how to dress. She looks better now. I ball her sometimes. Don't you want to ball? You're a far-out chick."

"No, I'm just depressed." My mother had been diagnosed by now with bipolar disorder. I wondered if I had it as well. Here I was in a strange city where I didn't know anyone, and I'd gone home with a stranger from a bar.

"By the way, George, have you ever been married?"

He had gone to college, and I hoped he had been married. It seemed things might be in my favor if he had been to college and been married.

"I was going to marry Mary Ann. Uh, but what's marriage? Some dumb piece of paper. Three days before the wedding, I told Mary Ann I wasn't going to marry her. She has our son. Listen, I won't pressure you. I had an operation down there, and nothing comes out. I'll let you feel the scar."

I didn't really feel frightened. Just wanted to go to sleep. Maybe

I felt flattered. "Where is your roommate?"

"He's not here," George said, and helped me into the bedroom.

"What is this?" I said, tapping a large object beside the bed.

"It's a heater. It stands between my bed and Harry's. It gives us privacy."

"Well, I'm getting into bed. I can sleep in my jeans and cowboy shirt. Where is the bathroom?"

"About ten steps across from the end of the bed. I'll leave the light on. And if you change your mind...."

George never touched me. When I woke up, I could see it was light outside. I made my way to the bathroom and to the shower. When I came out, George was snoring. "Wake up," I said. "I need to go to the airport and fly back to Tallahassee."

"Okay," George said. "Your thirty dollars will probably buy you a one-way ticket."

The airport personnel let George walk me up the metal steps to the plane, and he helped me find my seat. "You are a far-out chick," he said, and he kissed me on the cheek. "Come back and see me soon." I heard him walk up the aisle as I fastened my seatbelt.

When I arrived at my dorm in Tallahassee, my good friend Leigh and some other students and the dorm advisor were about to call the police and my mother. I had been missing for twenty-four hours. I pulled Leigh aside and told her what had happened.

"You may be depressed," she said.

Some years later, my psychiatrist diagnosed the George story as a manic episode. Combined with the depression I had exhibited, he diagnosed me with bipolar disorder.

My husband and I have searched for George on the Internet, but we can't find him. I treasure the cue ball that he gave me. I just wish I could tell him how much I appreciate his saving my life.

***

A few days after I returned, my friend Susan from high school called and woke me up one morning. I answered the phone and stood up right beside the bed. Susan said that her brother Mark had killed himself the night before. He had driven to the beach and parked at a picnic shelter. He took a piece of rope and formed a noose. After that, he threw the rope over a rafter and put the noose around his neck. Then he kicked the picnic table over, hanging himself.

Shocked. I told Susan I'd meet her in Jacksonville that afternoon.

It was incomprehensible. Mark had been president of his senior class in high school, captain of the football team, and voted best-looking male student. I couldn't help but think of the song "Richard Cory."

> "But I work in his factory
> And I curse the life I'm living
> And I curse my poverty
> And I wish that I could be
> Oh, I wish that I could be
> Oh, I wish that I could be
> Richard Cory."

Unfortunately, Richard Cory went home and put a bullet through his head.

How in the world could I help in this situation? We had Susan and her younger brother Scott and both their parents to console. I took the Greyhound to Jacksonville, and Momma gave me a ride to Susan's house. We went in her room and took turns swinging on her basket swing. It was a big basket her father had mounted above her bed, and it had soft pillows, and you could get in it and swing. Susan's mother came in and said she was glad some family and friends had arrived from the Midwest because they were not nearly as emotional as southerners.

"I can't believe Mark is dead," Susan said. "But why?"

"I don't know," I said. "I wish I could help you."

"I just want you to listen," Susan said firmly. And then she began to cry.

I felt terrible.

My mother and I went to Mark's memorial service. We sang the Cat Stevens song "Morning Has Broken" and for the rest of my life I would associate it with Mark. The family had a reception after the service which I thought was brave. Susan told me at the viewing the night before Mark had looked pretty good. She cut a lock of his reddish gold hair to keep. She said the mortician tried to cover up the caved in neck with a high-collared shirt but you could still tell.

My friend Mary Baine who was a psychologist said there is so much guilt after suicide rather than in suicide. She said perhaps the person who commits suicide must take some of that guilt with them. She also said that, after the death of a child, the parents often split up. Sure enough, Mark's parents divorced.

So, would Mother and Billy miss me if I committed suicide? I thought they would. But would they understand?

***

At Florida State University I had a series of liaisons in which I was searching for men to convince me I was attractive. The first one was Bob.

I put on a silky flowered outfit in my dorm one night and went to a party. It was dimly lighted in the room, and a guy named Bob took up with me. "You have a pretty face," he said. But I knew he couldn't see it very well due to the lighting. He asked me to go home with him, and I went. We rode in a car with some other people to his business fraternity. Once Bob saw my face in the light, he said "Oh" in that way my grandmother said "Oh." We got undressed and got into bed but he didn't put any pressure on me the first night. "What do I look like?" I asked in the smoke-filled bedroom.

"Good legs!" he exclaimed.

"What else?" I asked.

"A well-proportioned body," Bob said.

"And what about my eyes?" I asked holding my breath.

"No worse than a case of severe acne," Bob said.

What? I thought. I repeated his words in my head. "No worse than a case of severe acne."

His words were incredibly crushing. I got up and went into the bathroom. It was just a house bathroom with a toilet and a sink. I was sitting on the toilet when I heard the door open and a light switched on. "Oh, excuse me," a male voice said. But he took his time turning out the light and closing the door.

Bob had a motorcycle, a big Harley. He'd pick me up at my dorm, and we'd go riding without helmets with my long blonde hair streaming out behind me. Often, we went to a steak house and had a delicious meal. We progressed into a regular sex life and then I went home for the summer. Bob called me one day, but by then I liked Christopher in Jacksonville. That relationship went nowhere.

***

Next came Peter. He was an albino guy who wanted me to spend the night. He had a good friend named John who was normal. One night I went over to Peter's and might have stayed longer except he commented that his friend John had said, "Peggy is a really pretty girl, but how do you stand her eyes?"

I decided to go home. Since Peter was an albino, he didn't look normal, so why was he coming down on me? Could I possibly be attractive with all these remarks coming at me? I often thought of suicide.

Then there was a guy named Tom. He visited me in my dorm room. He was a sophomore and had been kicked out of the Air Force Academy for cheating after his freshman year. Nothing much happened in the dorm room, but when Tom came to visit me later in my new apartment it sure did. Tom grabbed my blouse and ripped it. I was so surprised I did nothing. Then I told him to leave and never come back, which he didn't.

I talked to my friend Leigh about all these relationships, and she said she wondered if I should see a therapist.

Chapter Ten

Lloyd, one of my former readers at Florida State in undergraduate school, and always a platonic friend, told me I had the crummiest taste in boyfriends. Besides, he said they were assholes for their comments about my eyes. Lloyd was visiting me in my apartment, and suggested that he take me to the mall and buy me a pair of sunglasses. He said I must wear them. For some reason, I had never wanted to wear sunglasses, but at this point, in January of 1976, I felt okay about taking this step. Maybe it would make me look better to prospective men and also on my new job.

One day soon after, Lloyd said, "I just met a nice guy named Bill who moved into our apartment complex. It might not matter to him that you're blind. He's a decent guy, and I can tell by looking at his face that he comes from good stock. I'm going to have the two of you over for a Coke."

So that Saturday afternoon Bill and I met at Lloyd's apartment. I had worn a sexy tube top and shorts. And, of course, my new sunglasses. I loved Bill's great baritone voice and, after he had spoken only a few sentences, I was hoping he would ask me out on a date. I was feeling emotionally stable.

"I told you about Peggy's accident," Lloyd said in his blunt, forceful manner. My heart sank.

"You did," Bill said in a level voice.

After a short silence, Lloyd asked Bill, "Weren't you in the Air Force?"

"Yes. I came to FSU for two years, went in the Air Force, and am now back here on the GI Bill, finishing my undergraduate degree in Finance. In the Air Force I tested high for languages and was sent to California to the Monterey Language School to learn Mandarin Chinese. Then I went to Taiwan for a year and a half as a military interpreter."

"How interesting," I said. "Glad you came back here to FSU. I finished my undergrad in English, June of '75. After that I just wanted a secretarial position for a year or so. I had to interview for 22 jobs before I got one. Somehow, I landed an interview in the office of the number two man in the Florida Department of Education. He said I deserved a job just like any sighted person. He asked if I could type from a Dictaphone, and I said I could. So, he placed me in an open secretarial position in his department. I don't think the immediate manager was too pleased, but she couldn't go against the number two man. So that is where I have been working for the last few weeks."

I hoped Bill liked me and would ask me out on a date. The twelve apartments in our complex all had the same floor plan. We were sitting in Lloyd's living room, which was designed exactly like my living room and Bill's living room. Unlike me, Lloyd had a coffee table between his sofa and chairs, where we placed our Cokes on coasters.

"Can I use your bathroom?" I asked knowing I knew exactly how to find it.

"Sure," Lloyd said.

"Do you need any help?" Bill asked.

"No, but thank you so much for asking," I replied. I wanted to show Bill how well I could navigate in a familiar setting.

I was delighted to cross that living room unaided—straight through the kitchen, which smelled like beer, and into the bathroom, which smelled like pee. Afterward, we talked a little longer and then Bill stood up to walk me to my apartment downstairs.

"Can I help you on the stairs?" he asked.

"Oh, I'll just run down," I said, again wanting to show how well I could navigate in familiar surroundings; I ran down barely touching the railing with my hand.

"You're something else!" Bill exclaimed when he caught up with me. Standing beside him, I was struck with how tall he was.

"How tall are you?" I asked.

"Six feet six," he said.

"Wow!" I exclaimed. I had always heard that tall men were very attractive.

At my apartment door, Bill mentioned he had read the biography of Robert Russell who, I knew, was blinded as a child and who, I also knew, became a successful college professor. It felt good that Bill knew something about blindness. Then he asked, "Would you like to go to Baskin-Robbins for ice cream tomorrow night?"

I felt elated and accepted.

"See you tomorrow," Bill said and patted me on the back. I tingled all over. Next time I hoped he would kiss me on the cheek.

After Bill left, I sped to the phone on my bedside table and dialed. "Leigh!" I shouted. "This really nice guy has asked me out for ice cream. He's very tall and was in the Air Force. I love his voice and… What did you say?"

"Oh," I continued, "your parents just got here from Jacksonville? Call me later."

Leigh was one of my best childhood friends. She was the first person I told about running away and staying with George.

In a way, Lloyd was right; I had had some crummy boyfriends. They all made fun of my eyes.

***

That night I tossed and turned. I wanted to call Bill, but I didn't have his phone number. Even if I had, I didn't think I should call him at one, two, or three in the morning. I hugged my new teddy bear, which I named Bill. Finally, my Braille watch read 7:00 a.m. Just twelve and a half hours until my date.

At work I felt like I was a million miles away. A couple of my coworkers pointed out that I sure seemed distracted. But I forced myself to focus. I knew my manager was not happy to have me there.

I valued my job. I tried to type my manager's letters from the Dictaphone perfectly. In those days, there were no computers and no screen-readers. It was a real challenge not to make a mistake, since I couldn't see what I was typing. Fortunately, I did quite well.

But I couldn't stop thinking about Bill.

I got home at 5:30 and took my second shower of the day. I blow-dried my hair and put on what I knew were light blue pants and a light blue silk blouse with bird-feather designs. Then I got cold, sweaty hands and wondered if Bill was coming. What if, after all, he didn't like blind people? Still, I sprayed on some perfume. Where were the sandals with heels? Finally, I found them under the bed. At 7:27 I was pacing the living room. I pulled out a strand of my long hair and nervously twisted it through my fingers. And then someone knocked lightly on the door.

When I opened it, Bill said, "You look very pretty tonight."

I was glad I had on sunglasses. Still, it was hard for me to thank people for compliments on my appearance. I said, "I like your aftershave."

"Thank you," Bill said.

"And I think it's cool you're so tall," I added. The more to love, I thought. "Hey, Bill, before we leave the complex, I need to show you the sighted-guide technique."

"What's that?" Bill asked.

"I'll hold on to your arm above the elbow as you guide me around. Keep your arm straight and relaxed. Don't run me into cars in the parking lot. If we're around steps, tell me when to step up or down."

We practiced in and around the parked cars and then got into Bill's MG. "Want the top down?" he asked.

"Maybe on the way back," I said. "I'd just like to talk on the way over, and it's harder to hear over the wind."

"What are your hobbies?" Bill asked as we drove along.

"I love to write, and I love to read," I said. "My favorite book is Steinbeck's *East of Eden*." I could as easily have mentioned Truman Capote's *In Cold Blood* or Dreiser's *An American Tragedy,* which were close runner ups.

"I love to read," Bill said. "My favorite book is *Once an Eagle,* by Anton Myrer." The title, he said, came from a Libyan fable, quoted by Aeschylus: "Once an eagle, stricken with an arrow, said, when he saw the fashion of the shaft, 'With our own feathers and not by others' hands are we now smitten.'"

I wondered if such an interesting guy would stick with me. I kept thinking about what my grandmother always said: "A handicapped man can marry, because a woman will marry anything, but a handicapped woman...."

"Where are you from?" I asked.

"Miami. Great place to play golf. One year I played 388 rounds."

"Wow!" I said. "My dad was a golfer."

Bill stopped the car and his keys jangled as he removed them from the ignition. He opened his door and a few moments later opened mine. I was thrilled I could hold on to his arm, could touch his skin below the fabric of his short-sleeved shirt. The January air was mild, even for Tallahassee.

"Let me know if the door to Baskin-Robbins opens in or out and on the right or left," I said.

"Glass door opening out to your right," Bill said. We made it through. Navigating strange doors can be a nightmare.

The ice cream shop was filled with conversations blending together. I knew people were staring at me, but at least I couldn't hear any whispered remarks over so many people talking. And, so what if they whispered? I was on the arm of a tall, sighted man. My heart sang.

"Do you want me to read you the thirty-one flavors?" Bill asked.

"I already know what I want," I said. "A double rocky road on a sugar cone, please."

Bill ordered mine, and he got a double strawberry in a sugar cone. We sat at a two-seater table. Bill's knees touched my knees, and I liked it. "The chocolate and marshmallows are divine," I said as I devoured my ice cream cone. It was hard to talk over all the conversations. I found it interesting that Bill had asked me so little about my blindness. In a way, I wanted to tell him all about the aspects of being the odd man out. Maybe I would tell him my tandem-bike stories and how fun that had been. Or maybe I'd just go out and buy a bicycle built for two.

After we finished, we got back in the MG. Before Bill turned on the motor, I said, "Maybe I'll buy a bicycle built for two."

"I'd love to go riding with you," he said. "You're such a pretty girl."

My heart raced, and I could not reply.

We drove along with the top down. The wind whipped my hair. I felt happy, which was unusual for me. Blindness and the disfigurement had been so hard, and then there was all the disappointment about Mother and Daddy. Happiness was indeed rare.

At my door, Bill kissed me on the head, but he didn't come in. What a gentleman! Soon I heard a very loud, very vigorous knock on my door. That was a "Lloyd" knock.

I opened the door and Lloyd said, "You didn't screw him on the first date, did you?"

"I most certainly did not, Lloyd," I said. "But I like him. Thanks for the introduction."

"Just checking," Lloyd said, and I heard his hard-heeled loafers walk away.

I sat on my sofa. A friend had helped me pick out the slipcover and throw pillows. The slipcover was soft and felt like velveteen. I knew it was yellow, and that the pillows were orange. I was thinking of long, tandem-bike rides. I knew there were some woods outside Tallahassee where we could find a shady place to kiss. What if Bill never called me again? I was raised to let boys call me.

And the very next day he called me at work. "Real quick," he said. "How about dinner and a movie Friday night? I'll whisper explanations of the silent parts of the movie."

"Great!" I said.

"I'll see you at 7:30," he said.

I hoped that, when he whispered explanations of the silent parts into my ear, maybe he'd give me a little kiss.

"Miss Paul," the manager said, "You don't seem to have your mind on your typing at all. What has happened to you?"

"She's in love," one of my coworkers said.

"You've been doing so well here," the manager said. "Please get your mind back on the job." But as she stepped away, I heard her laugh softly and say to herself, "But I was young once."

Back in those days, I had to do perfect touch-typing because there was no auditory feedback such as we have today with talking software. I actually managed to type a perfect letter before I went on to thinking about my outfit for Friday night. I had some new, light-yellow pants, and what I knew was a crisp white blouse with a red, yellow and black design. I asked a coworker if my gold earrings would look nice with that outfit, and she said yes.

I was ready at 7:15. At 7:30 there was a gentle knock on the door. It was Bill. He gave me a little hug. He took me, sighted-guide, to his MG. The pleasant weather had continued. When we got to the door of the steakhouse, Bill said it opened out and to the left. I touched the glass door and held on to Bill as we entered the restaurant. He had on a long-sleeved cotton shirt. My light-and-dark vision told me it was dark in the steak house. A band was playing. A waitress led us to a table, and Bill put my hand on the back of my chair. He got me seated, and I saw the flicker of candlelight in the middle of the table. Bill read me the menu, and I decided on a filet with rice and green beans.

The food arrived, and I tried to eat with care. My grandmother had always told me to use a biscuit to push with. Bill cut up the steak for me, but I ran into trouble with the rice. The waitress had not brought any bread, or a biscuit.

"I guess it's hard for a blind person to eat neatly," Bill said.

I was crushed. But without a biscuit or a roll, what could I do? I resolved to take eating lessons.

Bill said, "I didn't mean to hurt your feelings. I like you so, and I think you're so pretty. Let's finish up and go on to the movies."

I knew Bill was a very nice person. Still, I was sort of scared. I put my best foot forward, and we went to the movie. *Barry Lyndon* was long. We had Cokes and popcorn although I was already stuffed from dinner. The theater smelled kind of grungy—a combination of old cigarette smoke, greasy popcorn, and general mustiness. Bill filled in the silent parts and gave me a few light kisses on the cheek after whispering into my ear.

When we came home, he hugged and kissed me passionately for a while. I was on cloud nine except for the memory of the eating issue. All in all, I felt that Bill was starting to fall in love with me.

On Monday I called the visual-disability department at FSU and asked to speak to an activities-in-daily-living instructor. I asked her if she thought blind people had difficulty eating. She said, "No. I've seen a lot of fat blind people." I thought her remark was funny.

I said I was interested in the technique of eating neatly. So, she came to my apartment and gave me some tips. I've concluded that eating a sandwich in a restaurant is the best bet. You can control every bite.

I told my mother about Bill and asked her what she thought. "Whatever you think, sweetheart," she said.

I felt Momma was giving me more freedom.

I told my brother, who told my grandmother. Then my brother told me my grandmother thought Bill (whom she had not yet met) would milk me for all I was worth and then drop me. That reminded me of her expression "A handicapped man can marry because a woman will marry anything. But a handicapped woman…."

One day Bill and I got a ride to the bike shop. By this time, we had been dating for three months. It was early April, 1976. I bought what Bill described as a beautiful, silver tandem bike with black seats. I hoped—and I knew—we'd be riding lots of places.

I invited Bill to go to Jacksonville with me for Easter.

My grandmother called me the next day. When I picked up the phone on the dresser in my bedroom, she started right in. "I want to know if Bill is tall."

I laughed inwardly. "No problem, Grandmomma," I said. With Bill standing at six feet six, height was not an issue.

"Well, I have invited Tom and Teresa Palmer to go to Easter dinner with you, your mother, Bill, and me. I made a reservation at the Yacht Club for noon. I hope Bill has the appropriate manners for a country club. Tell him that when anyone other than the waiter or waitress comes to the table, the men stand up. Manners will get you through a powerful lot of situations. Anyway, do you have an Easter dress?"

"Yes, Grandmomma. I bought one the other day. Bill went with me to a dress shop at the mall to pick it out. He said the dress is a pretty shade of blue. The salesgirl picked out a blue-and-white scarf for me to wear with it, and I got a white purse and white shoes."

"Be sure to wear earrings, Peggy. Half the time you walk out all dressed and ready to go but without earrings."

"All right, Grandmomma. Someone is knocking on my door. It might be Bill."

"Oh, for God Almighty's sake," Grandmomma said and hung up.

Bill was at the door, and I invited him in. We sat on the soft velveteen cushions of the sofa. "My grandmother just called me, Bill.

She's worried that you're some kind of weirdo because you're dating a blind person. Why are you dating a blind person?" I asked.

"Because I'm falling in love with a blind person," he said, and kissed me on the head.

I couldn't believe it. I was thinking about the guys who had not called me after one-night stands. And here three months had gone by, and Bill was *so* interested.

***

Bill borrowed a car from a friend and drove us to Jacksonville for Easter weekend. It would have been a long tandem-bike ride. Then we went to the Yacht Club for the Easter buffet. At the table I felt the sterling silver forks and spoons, and what I knew was a white linen tablecloth. Bill said that each linen napkin was an Easter color: solid pink, solid yellow, or solid blue. Seated at the table were Grandmomma, Momma, Bill, me, and Tom and Teresa Palmer. Dr. Palmer had been both Momma's and my pediatrician. Everyone ordered a Bloody Mary or a mimosa. Already placed on our table, as I knew from past experience, was the best Melba toast and cheese spread I had ever tasted. The sound of Momma's knife scraping across a piece of Melba toast told me she was putting on the cheese spread. "Hold out your hand, Peg-a-roo, close your eyes, and I will give you a big surprise," she said.

"Thanks, Momma," I said and laughed as I ate the yummy treat.

As long as I could remember, Momma sometimes liked to say, "Hold out your hand, and close your eyes, and I will give you a big surprise."

My favorite surprise was a chocolate kiss or a glazed donut from Goodes Bakery. I wondered why my mother told me to close my eyes when she had a surprise for me in her hand. I couldn't see the surprise with my eyes opened or closed.

Bill offered to fix me a salad. I asked him to put everything on it except anchovies and to please give me a lot of black olives. When Bill stood up, Dr. Palmer said, "Bill, I'm glad you took your vitamins. Are you about six feet six?"

"Exactly, sir," Bill said.

Everyone but me left the table, and I fell into thought. My mother had grown up in a high-society Jacksonville family. After her divorce, she had to work as a schoolteacher to support us. Although Billy and I grew up with very little money, we had aunts, uncles and cousins who were very wealthy. Our grandmother took us to the Yacht Club to swim regularly as children. When we mentioned it to other kids in our middle-class neighborhood they said, "What's the Yacht Club?"

So here I was back at the Yacht Club, with its ballrooms, tennis courts, swimming pools, and boats nearby on the St. Johns River.

Bill's voice said, "Here's your salad, my dear," and I heard him set the plate in front of me. "I'll go get mine."

I hoped I would eat my salad neatly. I thought of all the food stations here: the omelet station, the roast-beef station, the ham station. And the salad, vegetable, and dessert bars. Soon the voices of my group returned, and the chairs scraped backward over the carpet.

"So, Bill, tell us about your family," Grandmomma said.

Let's grill Bill, I thought.

"My parents were from Michigan," Bill said. "My father graduated from the University of Michigan with an accounting degree. He worked for over forty years as an accountant and manager for GM. My mother was a housewife, and my sister works for Delta."

Hooray for the University of Michigan, I thought. Billy was finishing his second year of law school there.

"How did you wind up at Florida State?" Grandmomma said.

"Later in his career my dad transferred from Detroit to Miami. I spent some growing-up years there. Then I went to Florida State, left, went into the Air Force, and then came back to Florida State, where I'm finishing my degree in finance."

"Grandmomma, remember I told you when Bill joined the Air Force, he tested high for languages and was sent to language school to learn Chinese?"

"How interesting!" Dr. Palmer said. "Do you know Mandarin Chinese? Were you a military interpreter?"

"Yes, sir," Bill said. "I learned to read and write in Mandarin and was sent to Taiwan as a military interpreter."

"Then you're a very smart young man," Dr. Palmer said.

I heard the clink of the water pitcher touching our glasses as the waiter went around the table refilling them. As more and more people from the after-church crowd entered the dining room, I knew their voices would block such small sounds.

"Peg-a-roo, I see you have swept across your salad plate," Momma said. "Would you like me to get you an omelet?"

"Or I can," Bill said.

"Have you eaten any of your own salad?" I asked.

"I've had some. What kind of omelet would you like?"

"Mushroom and tomato," I said. "And, Mom, thanks for the offer. But you go ahead and get yours."

"This is a Lucullan feast," Grandmomma said. "Excuse me, but I need to go remind Addie Crosby about the book club meeting at my house this Thursday."

I automatically relaxed when Grandmomma left the table.

"You look pretty today, Peggy," Mrs. Palmer said. "I think this boyfriend agrees with you."

I smiled. I wondered if she would comment on my mother's beauty, but she didn't. I was relieved. I took a sip of my ice water. Soon I heard a plate being set in front of me. "Here you go, sweetheart," Bill said. I smelled what I knew would be a delicious omelet.

"Addie says to wish everybody 'Happy Easter,'" Grandmomma said. She was back at the table. "Addie looks older than the hills."

I looked toward what I knew was a wall of windows. I could see the sun was shining. I wished Bill and I could step outside for a moment and listen to the waves lapping on the St. Johns River.

***

A year later Bill proposed, and I accepted. For a while I put my left hand out to shake hands with people instead of my right hand. I wanted everybody to see my engagement ring. Grandmomma wanted us to marry at St. John's Episcopal Cathedral in Jacksonville, and she said she would pay for a high-society reception at the Yacht Club. I had the feeling that if I married in Jacksonville some of the people coming to the wedding would be coming just to see who would marry a blind girl. So, I told her I would have my wedding in Tallahassee. I had a lot of friends there who already knew Bill and wouldn't be curious about him. I also figured that anyone invited from Jacksonville who would come to my wedding in Tallahassee must really care about me.

Bill's father was in the hospital when we married, but his mother and sister gave a lovely rehearsal dinner at the Tallahassee Hilton. I wore a pretty, low-backed dress. Billy said Grandmomma kept speculating on what Bill's mother might really be like. It turned out that Grandmomma and Norine hit it off just fine.

***

That night I couldn't sleep. I was getting married the next day—August 20, 1977. What I kept thinking about was a minor scene after the rehearsal dinner. My friend Leigh, who was one of my bridesmaids, came up to me and drew a crisscross on my back with her finger. She said she could see the bathing-suit lines where the straps of my suit had blocked the sun. Over and over, I thought about the fact that I should have worn a dress with a high back. What was that—a defense mechanism? Distraction maybe? Focusing on something minor instead of thinking about on the major issue? Probably I was scared to marry, given that I was the child of divorce, and that I was marrying a sighted person. My head felt so uncomfortable in my hair rollers, but that couldn't be what was keeping me up. I slept in rollers all the time.

On my wedding day it felt like it was going to rain. Billy drove me to church in his old Volkswagen. He had just graduated from law school at the University of Michigan and was going to clerk for a judge in Texas for a year. On the way to the church, it started raining, and the sunroof leaked water on me. "But my hair!" I cried.

"You'll be wearing flowers in it," Billy said calmly.

"Do you think I look pretty, Billy?"

"You're not repulsive, Piglet," he said.

"My hair is ruined and it's your fault!"

"Calm down, Piglet, you've always been histrionic."

I forced myself to forget about my hair and think about something old, something new, something borrowed, and something blue. I had on my aunt's old pearls, my new white high heels, a borrowed wedding dress, and a blue garter. Billy was going to give me away. I wondered if Daddy was coming. His fourth wife was about to have a baby. At least Billy had an umbrella. We dashed into the church narthex. We found Grandmomma talking to a man who turned out to be Daddy, of all people. She hated Daddy, but for some reason she was being completely cordial to him.

"Hi, Dad," said Billy.

Before Daddy replied, Grandmomma said, "You are Ken Paul?" Then, "Oh..." And she stormed away.

No one has ever said the word "Oh" in a more scathing way than my grandmother said it to my father that day.

I wasn't very happy my father showed up either. I had no idea what he might say to me or to my new husband, or to any or all of the guests at our wedding.

"Peggy," Daddy said, "The wedding planner says you didn't have a boutonniere made for me."

"I'm sorry," I said. "I didn't think you were coming."

The rain was pounding harder on the roof.

At that point my two bridesmaids, Leigh and Judy, came up to hug me. The three of us stood for a moment in an embrace. I knew Leigh was wearing a blue dress that she had previously worn as her first wedding dress. Judy was wearing a yellow dress that she'd had made to match the style of Leigh's dress.

"Hi, Peggy," the wedding planner's voice said. "Where is your makeup?"

"I didn't bring any," I said. "People say I have a great tan."

"Well, your hair looked better last night at the rehearsal dinner. But at least you'll have the flowers in it."

I felt terrible about the wedding planner's remark. However, there was nothing to be done now but get married. And then I could go on my honeymoon with Bill. I stood with Billy in the back of the church waiting for the organ to play "Here Comes the Bride." When the first note sounded, Billy walked me down the aisle. Bill and I said our vows with the greatest sincerity. At the end of the service, everyone stood to sing "Joyful, Joyful We Adore Thee." I had chosen this hymn because I loved Beethoven, and the hymn was set to the melody of Beethoven's "Ode to Joy." Also, Momma had taught me the lyrics of "Ode to Joy" in German. Sometimes she and I sang the German together: *"Freude, schöner Götterfunken...."*

We had the reception in the church hall. As I stood in the receiving line and greeted each guest, I recognized the voices of many friends from Jacksonville and marveled that they had driven three hours to my wedding. We had invited 120 people and 115 came, including friends from Tallahassee. I really don't know what I talked to everybody about. I remember Bill fed me my first bite of wedding cake, and I fed him his first bite. Everybody chuckled. At last, Bill's best man whispered to me that he was going to drive Bill's car around. Bill came over, and his dark jacket felt so smooth.

My new mother-in-law made dainty little cloth packages containing rice. (In those days, rice was still thrown.) So, Bill and I made our way outside and were showered with rice. Bill helped me into the big old Delta-88 Oldsmobile he'd bought second-hand, and we drove away toward Myrtle Beach.

We honeymooned in a cottage on the beach. We delighted in each other, and on the surf and the sand.

One day, we went to a carnival in town where a carnival worker created anything you requested as a newspaper headline. We chose "Bill and Peggy Comin Honeymooned in Myrtle Beach."

We had the newspaper page framed, and kept it.

We moved to Charlotte, North Carolina in 1978. Bill worked as an industrial engineer for Burlington Textiles. I transferred into the Charlotte Junior League and enjoyed the volunteer work. Still, I wanted a paid job so I talked to my Junior League friends about it. One woman's husband got me an interview at North Carolina National Bank. I was very worried that I would not be hired because I was blind. But NCNB Human Resources called and said they wanted to offer me a nine-month paid intern position in the public relations area. I was 27 years old and on board! It was April, 1979. I called Momma, and she said, "Peach Cake, I have always known you could do anything!"

***

The weekend before I started the job, Bill and I visited some friends who had a farm outside of Charlotte. We went out there on a Saturday and the four of us drank a lot of wine.

At some point, I asked the husband, Marshall, if I could drive his truck across the farm land. Since he was drunk, he agreed. So, Marshall and I got in his truck with me in the driver's seat. The only problem was, I mixed up the accelerator and the brake. With Bill and Monty looking on in horror, Marshall and I took off like a wild horse across blackberry fields. Marshall screamed at me to hit the brake, and I finally figured out which pedal was the brake and did as he instructed. We came to a screeching halt, and soon Bill and Monty came racing up at top speed to make sure we were okay. We all had a great laugh about it, and I was thrilled to have finally driven a vehicle.

***

I liked my manager, John, at the bank. The only downside with him was he was going through a divorce and could be a pain sometimes.

But John also had a great sense of humor. Sometimes when I was unable to figure out which chair in his office to sit in, he would say, "Have a seat right here in the navy-blue chair." Of course, he and all the other men wore navy blue suits.

The PR Department focused on internal (lengthy newsletter), and external (news releases) communication and promotion. The woman in charge of promotion had, for example, an ice rink set up in the bank plaza that Christmas.

Bill dropped me off every morning in front of the 40-story glass bank building in the heart of downtown Charlotte. I made my way through the plaza and always stopped to touch "Il Grande Disco." This was a huge, elaborate sculpture in the shape of a disc. It was supposed to be eye-catching and had cost the bank three million dollars. When I reached the building, I had to navigate through revolving doors, always a challenge for a blind person. Then I walked to the elevators, pushed the button, and eventually made it to my desk on the fifteenth floor.

I wanted to overcome my blindness and be a successful employee. The first wrinkle turned out to be the number of people I had to meet and was supposed to impress. John said that Laura, an unpaid college intern, and I were going to spend a week at the *Charlotte Observer*, the local newspaper. I didn't particularly like Laura, and she was constantly taking me by the hand and saying things like "Let's go by the ladies' room." At these times, I didn't need to go to the ladies' room.

Laura and I sat in the lobby of the *Observer* and a lady, Marsha, whispered to her, "It must be so hard to be blind."

While I agreed with the comment, I hated for people to whisper, and I doubly hated for them to whisper about me.

At that point Laura offered me a piece of gum which seemed like a peace offering. I declined it.

After that, Marsha took us back to the news room. I had to hold onto Laura sighted guide which I hated. I wanted to walk independently.

We met a reporter named Carol Collier who talked to us about a story she was writing about Gloria Dunlap. Gloria was a young black woman in jail for killing her husband. The defense would be "battered woman."

Carol said she needed to tell us, two young women, something. She said male bosses expect their women employees to fail. She said we must educate our male bosses on this important point.

We then talked to an editor, Rich Oppel. He had a good deep voice and a strong handshake. As I stepped back from shaking hands with him, I ran into the side of his desk. I wondered if I would ever overcome these awkward embarrassments. I told Rich I followed his obituary controversy. He posed the question "Should we ever print anything negative about the dead?"

I told him all I wanted said about me was that I was wonderful.

Laura and I went to lunch with Ed Williams and Jack Jones. It was very awkward for me to figure out who to walk with, but I ended up walking with Ed. When we went back to the newsroom, I tried to find the bathroom and could not. Some guy named Joe rescued me and took me there. Laura came into the bathroom shortly afterward and said if she had known I needed to go, she would have helped me. I said aloud, "I want to be independent."

"Oh, butter, brickle, blond brownies," Laura said, presumably to lighten the moment.

I hoped my red linen skirt wasn't too wrinkled.

We went back to Rich's office and met a John McLaughlin who was visiting from the school board. He said it was important for editors to be human.

I liked the newspaper photographer we met named Frank. He had moved to Charlotte from Walla Walla, Washington. I was supposed to impress all these people and learn all their voices.

Next, we met Kathy, the movie critic. She said she had been thinking about how deaf people and blind people are cut off from movies. She said I should think about the fact that it was interesting for people to meet me because I lived in a different space. I wished she would talk to my manager, John. One time I didn't recognize someone's voice and he got really mad.

The next day I went down to HR to tell Mrs. Howie about how tired I was of going places with Laura. She said I should level with John and tell him I would make a better impression going to meet people on my own. For example, she said that Rolfe Neill, the publisher of the *Charlotte Observer*, would think I had guts if I stepped into his doorway alone. If I knew which wall to follow to his office door, I could do just that. Then Mrs. Howie gave me an inspirational tape. I took it back upstairs and started listening to it. The tape got all tangled up in the machine, so I asked a colleague to look at it. He said the tape was all screwed up, and it was probably a cheap tape anyway. Then he looked out his door and saw Mrs. Howie sitting outside. I was mortified, but Mrs. Howie seemed nonplussed that her inspirational tape was ruined. She said she didn't know where she had ordered it. I asked what I could do and she said, "That is your problem."

Blind people don't see people outside open doors. If I could have seen, I would have noticed Mrs. Howie immediately outside Jim's door. He was sitting behind his desk further back in the office so I didn't notice her at first. Not seeing people in the area is a real disadvantage. After the tape broke, I told the secretary I was going home for the day. On the elevator I thought about other situations where I had said something in front of somebody, and it was embarrassing. One day, my beautician told me she had a high-class call girl as a client. She said the girl was very obviously a high-class call girl. At another appointment, I said, "How's the hooker doing?" I thought my beautician would jab my head with scissors as she hissed, "She's in here right now."

On the bus home early from work, I began to think obsessively about the tape. I wondered if I could see, could I distract myself from this. I thought about how I ruined that tape, and how it must be irreplaceable, and how I was going to get into so much trouble with Mrs. Howie and the bank for ruining it.

My mind spun around and around. *How could I have ruined that tape? Why wasn't I more careful? Why did I borrow it in the first place? What was wrong with me? All I did was make mistakes?*

I tried to enjoy the cool air conditioning on the bus, because it was so hot outside. But it was hopeless. I knew I wouldn't sleep that night because I was so worried about the tape. Later in life I learned about psychological defense mechanisms. I understood that this kind of obsessive thinking fell under a psychological defense mechanism called distraction. In distraction we focused on something that is not really bothering us. Like the tape. That bothered me a little bit. I was really worked up about blindness and succeeding at work.

But I was like a dog with a bone about that tape. I stayed up all night obsessing over it, much to my husband's chagrin. The next day, one of the secretaries said she had found a place where we could order a replacement tape, and my colleague Jim asked me if I had really gone home because of that broken tape. I said I had, and he said he was worried about me and that it wasn't that big a deal. Jim actually learned how to write in first grade Braille on my Brailler. I really appreciated someone being that interested. That day he wrote: "What would you gain if you beat me with your cane?"

John did not understand how much energy it took for me to go out and meet a lot of people. He sent me to all these different areas of the bank, and some people asked me what happened to me. Typically, people asked, "Have you always been this way?" Which I interpreted to mean that the person wanted to know my story. The problem with all that was that I was blinded in such a horrible way. So, I usually just said I was blinded in an accident as a child. And then they wanted to know if I could see a little bit out of one eye and exactly how much I could see. And then they never could get straight what I could see or not see.

Meeting a lot of new people did not give me the opportunity to show what I could do in many areas. At least the people in my office noted that I learned to write news releases and that I wrote for the bank's internal newsletter. Best of all, I spoke well and was being groomed to be a public relations speaker for the bank.

So, I joined Toastmasters. Wikipedia defines Toastmasters as "a US-headquartered nonprofit educational organization that operates clubs worldwide for the purpose of promoting communication, public speaking, and leadership."

I was very successful delivering speeches, beginning with the icebreaker. In my speeches, I talked about growing up blind and related some of the funny things I had done.

***

Bill had been doing some training in computers in Charlotte, and he found a job he liked in that field in Atlanta. So, we moved to Atlanta in April of 1982.

We waited a while to have children. I knew they would be sighted, because there was no genetic component to my blindness. I wondered if I could handle children in that physically dangerous period between eighteen months and three years. Children at that point have mobility but no common sense. Two-and-a-half was exactly when I was blinded.

And then it happened—I got pregnant! The pregnancy flew by. My baby was due on August 21, 1983. In those days, doctors let expectant moms go two weeks beyond their due date before performing a C-section or inducing. It was September 3, and I was thirteen days beyond the due date. Bill and I went to a jazz festival in Piedmont Park, but it was cancelled due to rain. A minor disappointment, but it was the last straw. Bill said we had to cross a dirt path and cut through the grass to find a spot for our picnic. At first, I refused to cross. It was August in Georgia, and I was hot and tired and late in pregnancy. I was afraid to take on an unknown surface, both because I couldn't see it, and because of my lack of balance at that point due to the pregnancy. Bill explained that the path was dry, hard-packed dirt, and finally I agreed to cross.

The next day I awoke in the beginning of labor. I was in labor for only ten hours and was able to do natural childbirth. Bill and I had gone to Lamaze classes, and he was a great coach. At 6:17 p.m. on September 4, 1983, Meredith L'Engle Comin was born with her eyes wide open. I prayed she would have a long, wonderful and not-difficult life. Everyone said she was beautiful.

When Meredith was three days old, Mom came up and stayed in our apartment with us for a week. I was breastfeeding and exhausted. "Why didn't you tell me what it would be like with a newborn?"

"Some things defy description," Mom said.

During the day I kept Meredith in a playpen until she could crawl. Then Bill childproofed the apartment every morning before he left for work, and I let Meredith crawl everywhere all day. Mom had given me that freedom, and I wanted to pass it on to my children. When Meredith learned to walk, we did the same. I never lost track of her in the small apartment. I could always hear her somewhere.

One day when Meredith was a year old, I was sitting on the wooden rim of our glass-topped coffee table with Meredith in my lap. I leaned backward and the glass broke. We fell through, and I landed flat on my back on the carpet. I will never forget that terrifying sound of glass breaking. My baby! She had fallen through the glass with me and was lying with her head on my chest, her body on my stomach. What if she was cut or had glass in her eyes? But she was giggling, thank God. How was I going to get us out of there? My legs were still hooked over the edge of the coffee table. There must have been broken glass all around us, and possibly jagged pieces above us.

Somehow, I maneuvered Meredith through the wooden legs of

the coffee table and out into the living room. Then I pulled my own legs inward and struggled out of the wooden frame myself. At this point, Meredith was running around and still giggling. I realized my hand was bleeding. I picked Meredith up, carried her into the kitchen, and closed the door. I called Bill at work, and he said he would come home immediately. Meredith asked for some animal crackers, and I gladly gave them to her. She laughed out loud. Bill got home and checked Meredith out and said she was absolutely fine. Then Bill packed Meredith and me into the car and took us to Urgent Care to get a few stitches in my hand.

If Meredith had been seriously injured by broken glass, would it have been my fault? Absolutely. I don't know why we were so lucky.

***

When Meredith was 18 months old, we decided to buy a house. The apartment did not have a fenced-in yard for Meredith to play in, but the house did. We bought our daughter a sandbox and a swing set. Our ranch-style house also had two bedrooms, so we had one, and Meredith had the other.

When Meredith was two years old, we signed her up for preschool two days a week at First Presbyterian Church, near the Arts Center train station in Midtown Atlanta. Our house was located within walking distance of the MARTA line. Those two mornings a week, Bill drove Meredith and me to the church. While Meredith played in her class, I sat in an empty room in the church building and wrote, using my Perkins Braille writer.

At noon, I picked Meredith up, placed her in a backpack, and secured it on my back. Tapping my white cane in front of me, I made my way out of the building and turned right on the sidewalk heading for the MARTA Arts Center station.

"Train ride," Meredith called loudly from her perch. We listened to the beautiful church bells chiming hymns as we walked away.

Even with seasonal changes, I never remember a rainy day when we couldn't make this walk. Usually, the sun was shining; I could see its brightness and feel its warmth. Most of the time I stored my writing folder at the church, but on one particular day I had it in my left hand with my cane in my right. Just after I crossed 16th Street and stepped onto the sidewalk leading to the MARTA station, I dropped my folder. Three hundred pages of Braille fell out. At that moment it seemed that a breeze picked up. I stopped in my tracks and frantically wondered where all the pages were blowing. "Look at all the papers!" Meredith exclaimed. "The wind is breezing them."

And then I heard adult voices.

"I saw your papers flying around," someone said. "Here are twenty-five or thirty of them." Other people brought pages as well.

I was once again struck by the kindness of strangers. All of my papers were returned.

With renewed enthusiasm, I tapped my way into the MARTA station, turned right, stopped at the fare gate and fished my money out of my front pocket. I made it through with my cane and my daughter in the backpack. We descended two separate flights of steps. I tried not to inhale the smell of smoke and urine pervading the inside of the station. Down on the platform, I looked at the dark floor and then at the white strip signaling the edge of the track. I was grateful my mother had bought me a tandem bicycle and given me all the freedom she did. Otherwise, I would never have attempted to take my daughter in a backpack from her preschool class to the MARTA track. And then I heard it, the roar of the train we would board and ride home. We got on and rode to the station near our home. We got off there and walked home.

When Meredith was three, we bought her a nice rocking horse on a frame. She named the horse Cheyenne. To me, by the sound of it, Meredith rocked that horse very high. Bill confirmed visually that I was correct.

Every morning when Meredith got up, I fixed her a breakfast of Cheerios and orange juice. Then she jumped on her rocking horse. When she finished her ride, I gave her a small box of Sun-Maid raisins. Soon she brought the box back to me and said, "Mommy, I ate all the raisins."

I felt the box each day, and it was empty. One day I happened to take the cap off a pole of Cheyenne's frame, and to my extreme surprise, it was stuffed with raisins! So, Meredith knew she could put one over on her blind mother.

When Meredith was four, she got a new baby brother. He was born on December 4, 1987, and we named him Douglas Edward Comin. We rejoiced in his great health and, in fact, that we had two healthy children.

One warm, sunny day when Doug was eight months old, I carried him outside and put him in his fancy stroller, which was called a Maxi Taxi. I secured him with the lap belt and the shoulder harness. I double-checked to see that the stroller was locked in place. Then I dashed into the den and into the kitchen. I felt for Doug's bottle, which I had left to the right of the kitchen sink with the powdered formula already in it. I quickly filled it with warm water and raced back outside, shaking the bottle to mix the formula on the way. I put my hand in the stroller—and Doug was gone. I forced myself to remain calm. Bill was at work, and Meredith was at a friend's house. All the neighbors were at work. If Doug had crawled down the driveway, he could crawl right into the street and be run over by a car. If he'd crawled down the front walkway to the front porch, he might crawl up the steps—but he could fall back. I must have aged twenty years as I stood there wondering where he was.

Suddenly I wondered if someone had kidnapped him. Then something told me to walk the thirty feet or so toward the front porch. I put down my hand and felt Doug crawling up the steps. He was laughing. I picked him up and hugged and hugged him. Did I have a Houdini for a son? If Doug had crawled into the street and been killed by a car, would it have been my fault? Of course. I was the adult in charge of the child. But why do terrible things sometimes happen and sometimes not? I guess sometimes our guardian angels are around and sometimes they are on vacation.

Doug was a climber. Once he started walking, he climbed everywhere. He'd pull a kitchen chair up to the kitchen counter, climb up onto the chair, then climb up on the counter before I caught up with him. One time before he was two, he made his way up to the top of the refrigerator.

Another day, Doug crawled up on top of the washing machine, picked up the iron, stepped down on a chair, got on the floor, and plugged the iron in before I caught up with him. Much to my horror, the iron was already warming up!

The next morning, I told Bill I was going out for a brief walk before he left for work. It was early. I did not take my cane with me. It felt sort of misty outside. I walked along with my mind a million miles away. I heard a car coming. Surely, I had not crossed a street. I turned and ran into what I thought was a yard.

The next thing I knew, I had been thrown up into the air and landed hard on my hands. *What happened? Had a car clipped me?*

"You stupid idiot!" a man yelled. "You ran right in front of my car."

I stood up and thought I was okay. I motioned in his direction to go ahead. By then I had walked to safety on the grass. My neighbor, Mr. Stokes, said, "You took 20 years off my life, Peggy. I couldn't believe you ran in front of that car. I was sitting on my porch and jumped up. Are you okay?"

"I'm fine," I said. "I need to use my cane and be much more careful."

When I got home, Bill fixed me a cup of hot tea. We went on with the kids and the day, but the incident really scared me.

***

When Meredith went to kindergarten in 1989, she had an amazing first day. Doug and I walked her up to the bus stop in the morning, and she boarded the bus without hesitation. "There goes my Meredith," Doug said.

In the afternoon Doug was at a friend's house, so I walked up to the bus stop to meet Meredith. Other kids got off the bus but no Meredith. My friend Linda was there to pick up her daughter. We jumped into her car and literally flew to the elementary school.

"I can't find my daughter, Meredith Comin. This was her first day of kindergarten, and she did not come home on the bus," I said to the principal.

"Let me see what's happened," Mr. Hall said. In moments he added, "Oh, golly, she was put on the wrong bus. Go to the high school, because the bus driver will go there when he finishes his route."

Linda and I hurried to the high school. We went to the principal's office and found Meredith contentedly coloring a picture. "Hi, Mom," she said.

I scooped her up in my arms. "I'm so glad you didn't get off at the wrong stop, Meredith."

"Nothing looked like my stop," she said.

"Well," I said, "I'm going to make sure you are put on the right bus tomorrow."

"Okay," she said.

I've never heard of anyone who started out at kindergarten in the morning and made it to high school by the afternoon.

***

Once Meredith started kindergarten, I made a point of going to her school one day a year to talk to her class about blindness. I wanted to show the class what a blind person could do and answer questions in case Meredith or someone else had mentioned she had a blind mother. I visited Meredith's class from kindergarten through fifth grade, and Doug's from kindergarten through fifth as well.

I particularly remember the day I visited Doug's first-grade class. As always, I showed the students how I walked with my white cane. I also wrote each student's name on an index card in Braille. Then I brought out a copy of *Little Red Riding Hood*. It was one of the Twin Vision books I had for my kids. In this book, which was quite large, the print text and Braille text appeared on each page along with the storybook pictures. I read out loud to the class from the Braille text of *Little Red Riding Hood* and held the Twin Vision book up to show the pictures.

After that I explained that I would take questions, but that I could not see hands that were raised. I asked Doug to call on raised hands for me. I asked him to be sure to say the name of each child he called on, and not just to point.

First Doug called on Sara, and she had a question for Doug. Sara said, "Doug, can you get all the cookies you want out of the cookie jar since your mom can't see what you're doing?"

"No," Doug said. "My mom hears me open the cookie jar every time."

Then Doug called on John, who must have raised his hand. John said, "I like feeling my name in Braille. And I like your white cane. And *Little Red Riding Hood* is my favorite story. I want a blind mother!"

And then the kids chorused, "I want a blind mother, too."

***

Since both kids were established in school—it was 1994—I decided I needed a job. But first, I pursued a Master's degree in school counseling from Georgia State University.

The basic role of the school counselor is to support students in their psychological, academic, and social development. However, the breadth of school counseling is expansive. One minute the school counselor may provide a social-emotional lesson to a first-grade class, and the next they collaborate with the administrative team on a new schoolwide behavioral intervention system.

According to Heled and Davidovitch 2020, a school counseling role addresses the students' mental, emotional, social, and academic development.

School systems in various parts of the world have varying titles for school counselors:

Australia: student or education counselor
Bulgaria: pedagogical counselor
Denmark: pedagogical psychological counselor
USA: school counselor

In summary, the key elements of school counselor are:

–First, supporting the psychological, academic, and social development of students
–Second, resolving conflicts between all actors in school life
–Third, helping students face personal problems
–Fourth, consulting with students, parents, teachers, and principals
–Fifth, coordinating various school activities

***

After graduation, I was seeking employment. I participated in a number of interviews, but I was never hired. The county put me in a rotation for interviewing, and I participated in several, but I was never hired. Since I had a very high GPA and strong references, I could only conclude that I was not hired due to my blindness.

Then I decided to go into rehabilitation counseling. This meant another Master's degree from Georgia State. Part of overcoming my blindness involved a great interest in learning. It distracted me and made me feel equal to other knowledgeable people. In the end I focused on vocational rehabilitation.

To qualify for vocational rehabilitation services an individual must: according to the Website *Career One Stop*:

–First, have a physical or mental impairment that presents a substantial barrier to employment and be able to benefit from VR services to achieve employment.

–Second, need VR services to prepare for a job, or to get, keep or regain a job.

People who receive Social Security Income (SSI) and/or Social Security Disability Insurance (SSDI) benefits are considered eligible for VR unless they are considered too disabled to benefit.

VR is an individualized employment program. Participants may receive diagnosis and an individualized rehab program, counseling and guidance, training, job placement, and services to support job retention. Many applicants are referred by schools, hospitals, welfare agencies, and other organizations. Or, individuals may apply directly.

***

Usually, Meredith picked me up from Georgia State, but one day I took a taxi home. When the driver pulled into my driveway, he said there was a police car across the street from my house. I knew the teenager in that house was involved in drugs. I remembered I did not have a key, so I decided to go to my back deck and crawl in a kitchen window.

I took the screen off. I was pleased to find the window was not locked. I opened the window and crawled through. I was just about to jump to the kitchen floor below when someone tapped on my arm. "I am Officer Jones," a deep male voice announced. "Exactly what do you think you are doing?"

"I'm a blind person," I blurted out. "I live here."

"What?" he said.

Sometimes it was great to have blindness as an excuse. I didn't like being blind, but I didn't mind playing the blind card once in a while.

"Okay," Officer Jones said, "but I think it's kind of dangerous having a blind person crawling through a window."

***

Right after I finished my degree in rehab counseling, I got a job! I was hired by the Georgia Vocational Rehab Agency as a counselor. I soon passed my CRC which is the certification for rehab counselors.

I was assigned 100 clients with disabilities. My goal was to help them obtain jobs through training or education or help them retain jobs.

My clients included those with mental health disorders, partial paralysis, quadriplegia, autism, ADHD, personality disorders, stuttering problems, vision issues, and more.

Chapter Eleven

Next we had a role reversal. For many years, my husband had been there for me when it was time for medical appointments or eye surgery. Now, in 2007, he was the one who needed medical attention, and I had to see that he got it.

One evening not long ago, I arrived home from work on paratransit, made my way with my white cane to our driveway and hurried up to the back door. I expected to go in and call a greeting to my husband, who would be hard at work in his office. Instead, my sister-in-law met me in the kitchen and said, "Bill is in bed. He says the world is spinning around and around."

I flew upstairs. Bill was conscious, but he said when he opened his eyes, the world spun around. Then he threw up.

I called the doctor and reached the after-hours answering service. A nurse practitioner called me back and suggested we take Bill to an urgent care center or to the emergency room. Yet, at his recent physical, all his vital signs had been good.

After my sister-in-law went home, I called our adult children and told them I thought I would just let Bill rest overnight. Our daughter, who lives out of town, offered to come. Our son, Doug, who lives in town, told me he would be over at six a.m.

Bill fell asleep as I sat beside him. That's the way Doug found us when he arrived the next morning. When Bill awoke, the world was still spinning, and he still felt nauseated. I was worried he might become dehydrated. Doug and I decided to take Bill to the urgent care facility, but Bill could not walk. How could we get him down the stairs? I called 911.

The ambulance came with sirens blaring. The neighbors popped out to see what was going on. An emergency medical technician named John went upstairs to talk to Bill, who was fairly coherent. Another EMT named Jim asked me to go with him into the kitchen. Dim light came through the windows, but he asked that I turn on the ceiling light. I flipped the switch and explained that I was blind. My racing mind was distracted for an unreasoning moment to register relief that I had put the dishes in the dishwasher.

Jim called the fire department and asked them to bring a stair chair to get Bill down to the first floor. Then he asked me questions about Bill's health, and I signed paperwork. Our son, Doug, told me that he had to leave for work. I asked if I would be allowed to ride in the ambulance with Bill? Jim said I could. Doug handed me Bill's wallet. Then Jim helped me outside and into the front seat of the ambulance.

John and the firemen loaded Bill into the back. John said Bill's blood pressure was normal in the house but spiked in the ambulance, which was to be expected under stress. He put Bill on an IV for nausea.

It was so strange for me to take Bill to the hospital. For nearly four decades of marriage, he had taken me to Emory University Hospital for eye surgery—he drove there, handled parking, backed me up when I talked to doctors, and sweated it out when I was in the operating room.

I asked Jim, the EMT who was driving, what he thought was wrong with Bill. He said he and his partner thought it was "acute vertigo." While we talked, the ambulance radio was filled with reports of gunshot wounds and babies about to be born in cars.

At last, Bill and I were in a single room in the ER with a curtain for a door. Bill was transferred from a stretcher into a bed. "The world is still spinning," he said.

I texted the children to let them know we were in the emergency room. The admitting nurse came in. I pulled out the insurance cards and told the nurse I was blind. She took Bill's vitals, said they were normal, and asked me a number of questions about Bill in regard to heart disease, cancer, and stroke. Seemingly, the man was in great health. I signed more paperwork.

Soon the doctor walked in and diagnosed Bill with acute vertigo. She ordered bloodwork, an EKG, and an MRI of the brain in case a stroke was involved. I knew from my job as a rehabilitation counselor that most strokes were caused by high blood pressure, but some could be brain related. The doctor asked the nurse to hook Bill up to IVs for fluids and more anti-nausea meds. She said she was debating between including Antivert in the IV or Valium, either of which could treat the vertigo. I almost jumped up and said, "Please give Bill the Antivert, but give me the Valium!"

She did give the Valium to Bill, and he said the world stopped spinning almost immediately. He got so relaxed he started recounting episodes from *Doc Martin*, a wacky comedy series about a socially inept small town British doctor.

Bill's blood was drawn, and a cardiac tech did an EKG. An MRI tech came to take Bill away for the test, estimated to last about 25 minutes. I walked back into the huge emergency room with my white cane. A woman asked if she could help me, so I asked her if she could take me to a bathroom. When I emerged, I received another offer of help from a second woman and asked her if she could take me to the cafeteria, where I quickly downed a BLT and a Coke. My newfound friend waited for me and took me back to Bill's room just as he arrived there.

The doctor returned soon after and said Bill had a beautiful brain, a normal EKG, and normal blood work. She referred Bill to an ear, nose, and throat specialist and said he would come out of the vertigo as quickly as he had gone into it. She handed me three prescriptions to have filled. Then, after five hours in the ER, Bill could go home.

So, now we had a blind woman and her incapacitated, sighted husband trying to figure out a way to do that. Fortunately, our son soon arrived and drove us there. The next day, Bill and I walked three miles, and he drove me to the grocery store. Four days later, Bill took me to Emory for laser eye surgery. The roles had switched back.

But somehow things had changed. I now realized that Bill was vulnerable. We hoped the ear, nose, and throat specialist would find the cause for his vertigo, but a lot of tests still had to be run. What if Bill had frequent episodes of vertigo? Would he lose his job? Would I have to quit my job to care for him? What would happen to us financially?

Yet the strongest feeling I had was an overwhelming love for my husband. I thought about the vows we had taken many years ago: "For better or worse, for richer or poorer, in sickness and in health." I knew that whatever happened with Bill's health, I would figure out a way to handle it.

Chapter Twelve

In 2008, when I was fifty-five, my ophthalmologist, Dr. Doyle Stulting at Emory Eye Center, told me I might regain some vision with a corneal transplant. He said that such a procedure could succeed at last because of steroids. Of course, only my left eye was operable, and only some of the vision in that eye might be regained. Still, that was exciting news, and Dr. Stulting said he would do his best.

Bill took me to Emory on the appointed day. The techs and nurses prepared me for surgery. The anesthesiologist put me in twilight sleep, and Dr. Stulting performed the transplant. I was alert enough to hear him give a few heavy sighs, when he did the fine stitching attaching the new cornea to my eye. Once I was fully awake, I touched my face and felt the metal shield he had secured over my eye with bandage tape. I went home the same afternoon with his instructions to leave the shield on for 24 hours.

When I removed it the next day, I looked at the stovetop in our kitchen in Atlanta. Immediately, I knew I could see better. Those dark circles must be burners! I touched them and confirmed that they were. I walked to the kitchen table. I saw a small, light item and a small, dark item. I touched them: one was the salt shaker and one was the pepper shaker. I saw a much bigger light-colored item. I picked it up and found it was a paper napkin. I tossed it on the kitchen floor. The paper napkin made no sound. But I saw the light color of the napkin contrasting against the dark of the floor and picked the napkin back up. What a miracle! I walked over to the kitchen sink and saw things in it. Oh, no! Those must be dirty dishes.

The mind has no picture of what it has never seen. The tactile has to be transposed into visual through thought.

My adult children showed me an image of a kite in a picture book and asked me what it was. I had no idea. When they said it was a kite, I recalled what a kite felt like and then transposed that feeling into the shape I saw on the page.

I learned to read very large print letters. I already knew what letters felt like because my mother had given me many ABC blocks with raised letters on them when I was a child. I studied and learned print visually at the age of fifty-five. Again, I had to transpose the tactile into the visual. I started slowly to read newspaper and magazine headlines. One day, while waiting to see Dr. Stulting at Emory, I read the following magazine headline: "Water Wars Pitting Farmers Against City Dwellers and State Against State."

I loved to hang out at grocery stores and read the large-print names on cereal boxes. Sometimes I did a dance of delight in front of the boxes. Often my husband just dropped me off on the cereal aisle while he did the grocery shopping.

Another great joy for me was learning colors. I knew red, but Bill took me to the paint store and showed me every shade of blue, green, yellow, orange and purple. One day I was looking at a travel magazine and saw the word "Beijing," on a beautiful blue background. I decided my new favorite color was blue.

Contrast was important, and I learned to write with a black marker on white paper. I printed many notes to family, friends, and colleagues. Best of all, they could read them.

While I still read from my computer at work using JAWS (Job Access With Speech), a screen reader, I also tried to master ZoomText, a software program that magnifies print letters. Because I had only recently learned to read print, I was very slow. I just wasn't fast enough to benefit from large print on the computer screen.

In the Freedom of Space

In my job as a vocational rehab counselor for the Georgia Vocational Rehab Agency, I had to do a lot of work on the computer. JAWS read every word, every line, every sentence, and every paragraph out loud so I could hear my work. Much of it was also done with clients interpersonally. The mission of our agency was to help people with disabilities become competitively employed.

I worked in the lovely Marietta office. Once I learned colors, I would stare at the beautiful blue walls and orange walls that defined the interior office space. The colors gave me visual cues as to where I was.

I loved to go outside into the parking lot. If I saw a big blue or yellow or red object between white lines, I knew it was a car. If there was no car, I loved to jump over the white lines. I also loved to go to the sidewalk and look for the dark cracks in the white cement and jump over them. What was the saying, "Step on a crack and break your mother's back?"

Momma was thrilled about my new vision, but she seemed very skeptical about it lasting. I reveled in my new found freedom and knew that Momma had put me on the path of freedom with gifts like the tandem bike.

On the first day in my office with my new vision, I sat at my desk and saw a blue object. It proved by feel to be a stapler. I saw and felt other objects which proved by feel to be a black tape dispenser and a brown staple remover. The immediacy of vision allowed me to pick up an object without feeling all over the desk for it.

I also noticed the dominance of vision. With our ears we hear a few sounds, like the dryer running in the kitchen or some music playing, but with our eyes we can take in so many things at once.

My new vision was limited, but it was very exciting to me. Even with the corneal transplant, I couldn't see faces clearly. People always bemoaned the fact that I couldn't see the faces of my husband and or my children. I knew them by voice and personality, and by the feel of their hugs. When I hugged Meredith, I felt her petite frame and silky hair. When I hugged Doug, I felt his tall athletic frame and coarser hair.

Interestingly, I could pick out more facial detail on a television screen than on a real person. Perhaps it had something to do with the lighting. At times I stared at what must be a face and heard the voice of a female news anchor. I could see her eyes blinking, her head turning, and her mouth moving. Somehow, for most of my life, I'd had the idea that a person's face must look the way a doll's face felt: inanimate and still. I couldn't believe all the motion in the TV face.

Close up and in person I could see some gestures. These fascinated me. I could not believe how much people gesture and how much it adds to a conversation. "Thumbs up," "A-okay," "Fingers crossed," "I give up," "Hooray!" "Hands folded in contemplation," "Stop!"

I tried to learn to wave, but my daughter said I waved like a beauty queen. My son watched all my antics and said I was like a kid in a candy store.

Dr. Stulting said I would never drive or read small print but that he was cautiously optimistic that the gain in vision would last.

Bill took me to the zoo. We went to see an elephant. I stared. "Why didn't you ever tell me about the *size* of an elephant?"

"How do you describe the size of an elephant?" Bill replied.

Next we went to the petting zoo. I touched a sheep and then a cow. I could not believe that a cow was taller than a sheep. Again, I stared. Blind people have many incorrect perceptions.

Next we saw a bottle-nosed dolphin in its tank. As I watched, the dolphin swam gracefully upward. When I think of grace as a picture, I think of a dolphin swimming gracefully upward.

On the way home, we stopped and watched some koi fish swimming in their tank. I saw them zip by at the highest speed. Then they clustered together as if they were having a meeting.

***

The new found vision only lasted a few years. The cornea rejected, and I was back to light, dark, and red.

Momma had protected herself and didn't seem surprised.

My husband and my children and my brother were heartbroken, as was I.

Chapter Thirteen

The Now

Momma, age eighty-six, and I, age sixty, were sitting on the wonderfully comfortable sofa in the living room of her cottage. It was early morning. I touched the soft fur of Jenny, the cat, who was lying between us. A blue jay shrieked outside and another blue jay responded. Jenny didn't make a move.

"Mary Ruth is preaching this Sunday. Her text is from the book of Isaiah. She is such a superstar here from growing up in that Japanese internment camp."

"You're a lovely person, Momma."

"I'm nothing. The people here at retirement center are involved in all kinds of ministries and volunteer activities. Florence is always doing good works and is such an angel."

When Momma asked me to talk to her psychiatrist about her case, he shared important information with me. He told me she projects her insecurity onto other people, and there is nothing he can do to change it. I asked if that led to jealousy and low self-esteem, and he said it did. I also asked if I should encourage her to think positively, and he said no. At her age, he said she could not help thinking negatively.

I sat back further into the comfortable old sofa. It had been recovered at least three times during my life.

"Hold my hand," Momma said. "Let's talk about the good times we had. Remember when we went to Goldhead State Park and rode the paddleboats?"

"Yes, Momma."

"Let's play 'hum and guess 'em.'" She started humming a tune.

"Molly Malone!" I cried out.

"That's right," Momma said. "And you do think I was the best mother for you?"

Here I had a problem. I loved my mother. I blamed her for my blindness but thanked her for my freedom. "Of course," I said. "Of course, Momma."

"Tell me you love me."

"I love you, Momma."

"Tell me again," she said.

"I love you, Momma. I'll hum a tune now."

But before I did, I wondered why Momma hadn't scooped up a little two-year-old and hugged her tight until the plumber was gone. How many of us expect a plumber to come into our home in the morning and blind our child for life before he leaves? At that point, I started to sing, "'Tell me why the stars do shine, tell me why the ivy twine, tell me why the sky so blue…" and at the last second I hummed it. Momma guessed it right away.

Then Momma hummed, "For All the Saints Who From Their Labors Rest," and I got it.

Then I hummed "Beneath the Cross of Jesus, I Fain Would Take My Stand." And she guessed it.

"I want to die sometimes," she said. And she hummed, "'When I Survey the Wondrous Cross on Which the Prince of Glory Died."

I guessed it right away.

"I want to sit here quietly and read my Bible for an hour," she said. "Let me know if you want me to read you some psalms."

I said, "I'll just sit here and think."

I looked outside and saw the light of the sun. Light, dark, and red were all I could see. Except for my first two years as a child and a few brief years as an adult, they were all I had ever been able to see. I looked into the corner of Momma's living room at the red wingback chair. I loved the color red, because I could see it. I remembered my red rubber rain boots, red construction paper, my red car coat, my Barbie with the red velvet coat and red velvet hat, my silky red blouse I wore in the park, and a red dress I wore to make a speech at Wheaton.

"I'm going to read the Sermon on the Mount," Momma said, interrupting my thoughts. "Would you like me to read it to you?"

"I'm just thinking, Momma," I said.

"Meredith okay?" she asked.

"Fine. She's still working in digital advertising and also serving as a community vice president in the Cincinnati Junior League."

"And how is Doug?" she asked.

"He's fine, too. He is doing well as a paralegal at King and Spalding. And he does long-distance race biking on the weekend. He and his friends will bike 100 miles on Saturday."

"They are such sugar lumps," Momma said.

Jenny flopped back down on the sofa between us. I heard her purr. When she stood up, I heard her padded feet hit the bare tile floor.

Jenny meowed at the front door, wanting to go out. A blue jay shrieked. I looked toward the light. I turned my head in the direction of the wingback chair. Now, five years after the transplant, I once again could see only light, dark and red. I really missed the newfound vision I had enjoyed for the last few years. But my body had eventually rejected the cornea, returning my vision to what it had been after my childhood accident.

I wanted to say aloud, "Oh, Momma, can't we talk about it all? *Why* can't we talk about it all? We just have to talk about it!"

But, of course, I knew she could not. She couldn't talk to me about the horror of that day. She had built an impenetrable wall. She couldn't take it down so we could discuss the agony it had caused us both. She had sent me to a school for sighted children. This decision was incredibly unusual at that time, but she knew I would have to live in a sighted world. She had stood by while I negotiated my way out of my brother's wrestling holds. She knew that, as a blind person, I would have to keep my wits about me. She let me climb trees and bought me a tandem bike when I was ten years old. She'd told me I should ride on the back, only pretending to herself that I would obey. Shocked neighbors called her and said they could not believe they had seen her blind child steering the bike down major avenues while a sighted child rode on the back. Momma just thanked them for calling and did nothing. And at last, I understood the juxtaposition.

It was not for a lack of love or attention on her part that she let me do these things. I believe I had so much freedom because she planned for me to have it. Of course, because of her depression, she sometimes lacked the strength to reel me in when I took it too far. At times, the best she could do was lie in bed, smoking cigarettes and reading novels.

A beautiful line from Viktor Frankl came to me. He drew it from Psalm 118: "I called to the Lord from my narrow prison, and he answered me in the freedom of space."

It was the space of the outdoors and the wind that blew by me as I roller-skated and rode the bike that gave me life. It was the freedom the outdoors provided that made me live.

My mother and I would always be locked in a narrow prison in which we could not talk about the day I was blinded—but God had provided Momma the wisdom to raise me in the freedom of space!

www.ingramcontent.com/pod-product-compliance
Lightning Source LLC
LaVergne TN
LVHW051835080426
835512LV00018B/2882